"The incredible *magia* of Laura Davila's book, *Mexican Sorcery*, doesn't come just from her meticulous research but also from decades of lived experience. In this no-holds-barred deep-dive into the landscape of Brujeria De Rancho, Laura guides us through important history, powerful spells, and necessary truths with clear and gentle honesty. Never before has there been a brujeria book written in English that contains so much heart and soul. This is the book that will change the magical community's understanding of our *magia* forever."

—J. Allen Cross, author of *American Brujeria*

"Laura Davila's work perfectly reflects the Brujeria de Rancho in Mexico, one that transcends borders despite her being born on this side of the river. Her book is powerful like cacti, full of magic like the night in the desert, and spicy like the chili that burns in the candles on Good Friday. Laura is a ranch witch by birth, heritage, and will, and an excellent exponent of real witchcraft in northern Mexico."

—Paola Klug, author of *Relatos de las Brujas Morenas* and *Grimorio de las Brujas Morenas*

"Thank you, Daphne la Hechicera, for providing an excellent book that offers accessible magical rites, and showcases the beauty and eclectic nature of Brujeria de Rancho. Along with her diverse magical recipes, she brilliantly interweaves tales, stories, and Mexican folklore. I loved this book!"

—Erika Buenaflor, MA, JD, author of *Cleansing Rites of Curanderismo*

"Folk magic is about working with what you have where you are to get what you need (and sometimes, what you want). Laura Davila's book, *Mexican Sorcery*, shows you all this and more while maintaining a salty, sincere sense of humor that makes it a rare find on magical bookshelves. Her discussion of Brujeria de Rancho, Mexican-rooted rural folk magic, is a frank and sharp-witted introduction to her practices in their cultural context. She emphasizes how much this magic is both woven into daily life through the use of powders and prayers, and how special it is in reaching into the spiritual realm to solve problems outside the reach of mortal hands. She invokes the spirit of Chavela Vargas early on, noting that Mexican folk magic is about a sense of identity and that its power derives from the many threads of Mexican history across time. Davila gives you everything, no holds barred—from recipes for the *capirotada* dessert served at Eastertide to powerful *polvos* designed for use in the intense love-domination spells known as *amarres*. This is a book and an author who hold nothing back, and anyone attempting to learn about Mexican folk magic should be eager to learn from Davila's work."

—Cory Thomas Hutcheson, author of *New World Witchery*

"Laura Davila has written an outstanding book on my favorite subject: the tried-and-true sorcery born of necessity. Magic that, like love, transcends all time and space. The souls of the oppressed live in her every word. Their presence gives a bittersweet weight to her words without weighing them down. This book is about magic, but, most of all, it is about resilience and family and the ties that bind us in eternity. There are only a handful of books I have read that permanently reside in my heart. *Mexican Sorcery* by Laura Davila is now one of them.

—Mary-Grace Fahrun, author of *Italian Folk Magic*

"Laura Davila manages to take brujeria, a rarely publicized topic, and make it both easily digestible, as well as detailed. Many of the workings mentioned in this book I remember seeing my abuela do growing up, although she didn't know much about where they came from. Even today if you asked her about it, she couldn't tell you why she did them, it just simply *was. Mexican*

Sorcery touches on topics of Mexican folk magic that many people, including myself, have questions about but don't know where to look. For anyone interested in Mexican folk magic, this book will become a staple."

—Robyn Valentine, creator of Tired Witch, author of *Magickal Tarot*

"A meticulously researched guide for the seeker of Mexican folk magic, Laura Davila's *Mexican Sorcery* explores the folk Catholic aspects of this *magia* (magic) from a perspective grounded in history and founded on authentic practice. With its practical approach to Brujeria de Rancho, *Mexican Sorcery* is a valuable resource for any modern practitioner."

—Alexis A. Arredondo and Eric J. Labrado of City Alchemist, authors of *Magia Magia* and *Blood of Brujeria*

"Laura Davila presents the authentic magic of our *cultura* in an authentic way approachable to both experienced workers of Mexican magic as well as non-Latinx folks wanting a better understanding of how we do things in the *ranchos*. Abundant in cultural history, Davila sheds light on this extremely effective yet often overlooked magic of our Mexican culture. Encompassing health, wealth, love, and more, Davila reveals and gives cultural insight into how the pragmatic magic of our rural Mexico can be authentically adapted by anyone who truly intends to learn its secrets."

—Tomás Prower, author of *La Santa Muerte*

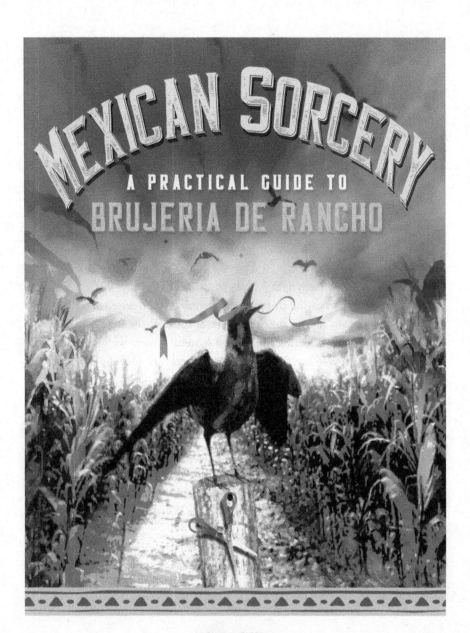

MEXICAN SORCERY

A PRACTICAL GUIDE TO
BRUJERIA DE RANCHO

LAURA DAVILA
daphne la hechicera

WEISER
BOOKS

This edition first published in 2023 by Weiser Books, an imprint of

Red Wheel/Weiser, LLC
With offices at:
65 Parker Street, Suite 7
Newburyport, MA 01950
www.redwheelweiser.com

ISBN: 978-1-57863-781-2

Library of Congress Cataloging-in-Publication Data available upon request.

Cover design by Sky Peck Design
Interior photos by Laura Davila
Interior by Steve Amarillo / Urban Design LLC
Typeset in Bely and Vintage Whiskey

Printed in the United States of America
IBI
10 9 8 7 6 5 4 3 2 1

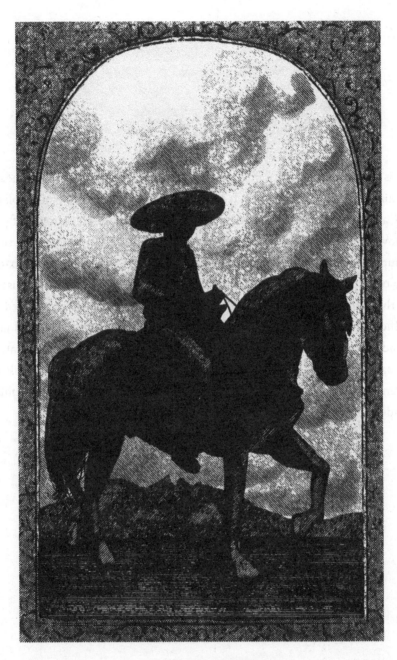

El Charro Negro by Jens Friborg

To all the mothers, grandmothers, and caregivers; the ones who dreamed us into being; the ones who have kept traditions, rituals, faith, and Mexican magic alive and who keep nurturing our culture and our souls; the ones still guiding us and protecting us, some of them still weaving their magic here on earth; others like mine from another realm; to your grandmothers, the ones like me who had to emigrate to give their kids a better life, the ones who were silenced, the ones who were not able to visit Mexico again due their immigration status, those who left part of their souls over there; to the ones who had to embrace a new language and a lot of times couldn't find the words to transmit the knowledge; to the others that we didn't get to know but are deeply rooted on our collective whispering like the wind so we do not forget and keep maintaining Mexican magic alive.

To my *abuelas*, Diana y Socorro, who taught me that magic and faith can open every door and some windows as well; to my *Abuelo el Profesor*, Raúl Oriente; to my *Muertos*.

To my husband, Scott, who has always believed in me and my magic. Scott, you did not let me forget who I am. You stood by my side each and every day, and every night, even in the darkest ones. You made sure I did not give up on my dreams, in my magic. You built me up, and did whatever it took to bring me back to my soul purpose. I am so thankful for you, my love. You are forever in my heart.

To my children: Pato, Manuel, Raúl, and Neil.

To my parents, Jaime y Laura gracias por darme la vida y la libertad de hacer con ella lo que he querido y verlo con buenos ojos.

My siblings and best friends, Marcela and Jaime, I love you guys. Thanks for always being there.

To Victor, my stepfather, for opening the doors of his house and welcoming me like a daughter when I arrived in the US.

I would like to extend my appreciation to Mariano Cabrera, alchemist by profession, and his invaluable help; Paola Klug for being a constant source of empowerment, inspiration, and help and who is today one of the best teachers of traditional Brujeria in Mexico. To J. Allen Cross, for believing in me, for encouraging me, for giving me that sense of belonging, for growing our community, and making a space in it for me. To Judika Illes and Weiser Books.

To the ones who feel oppressed, powerless, left out, the ones who live in fear due to their immigration situation, to our community, this is for you, thank you!

Cuando las mazorcas hayan crecido regresaras a este lugar
y dejaras otras semillas donde hallaste estas; es así como el
conocimiento se expande, tu recibes y a cambio das.

When the corn cobs have grown, you will return to this place
and leave other seeds, where you found these ones; This is how
knowledge expands, you receive, and you give in return.

—Paola Klug "Hombre Lluvia"
from *Relatos de Las Brujas Morenas*. My translation.

CONTENTS

INTRODUCTION

I am.
I am a part of each, and every one of them,
I am the seed, of my ancestor's seed, which has all their traits, their
    wisdom, folklore, their traditions, their faith.
Tlaloc on a rainy night.
Saint Michael's sword on an uncertain day.

—Daphne

El que nace para maceta no sale del corredor—This *dicho* (saying), which roughly translates to "the one that is born to be in a pot does not go beyond the corridor," refers to the fact that each person occupies a place for which they were born or for which they have been prepared for their entire life.

My immigration story is not a happy story. It was full of pain, sorrow, and grief, but without it, I probably would not have realized who I was, not only as a person but also as a *bruja*, a witch.

Bruja is not a nice word where I came from; people even bless themselves three times after hearing someone say it. When I was young, I was very naïve, and despised all the magical knowledge the previous five generations of my family gave to me on a silver platter. I was not ready for that to be exploited and celebrated. I did not know how to deal with judgment. I was not ready to be the witch, the bad one in someone else's story. Instead, I became the good victim, a victim of other people and my own circumstances. But then, when

I emigrated to the US, I had no other option but to be who I was destined to be. At that moment I finally made peace with my destiny in the place where I ran away to avoid it.

My name is Laura Davila, but in the magical world I am known as Daphne la Hechicera. I was born and raised in Monterrey, Nuevo León, Mexico and I emigrated to the United States twelve years ago. It was a couple of weeks before my twenty-fifth birthday. I spent the first seven years of my life in a big rancho in Rio Bravo, Tamaulipas, six minutes away from the border. My paternal grandparents' ranch had a cornfield and animals. It was full of nature spirits and absent of things like car horns, sirens, traffic, and city lights in the evening, allowing me to watch the stars every night.

That ranch is the reason why I refer myself as a *"bruja de rancho."* Bruja de rancho is an expression that was and still is used to refer in the rural areas of Mexico. Ranchos in Mexico are rural tracts of land, usually *ejidos*—areas of land held in common by the inhabitants of a Mexican village and farmed cooperatively or individually. Ranchos are used to plant crops and raise *ganado* (cattle), horses, goats, and sheep.

Many brujas de rancho were visited for services such as healing, divinatory, and advisory work. They even provided justice in cases where it was needed. La bruja de rancho has always been very iconic—especially for me—a figure to honor, redeem, and empower. Despite being rejected by Roman Catholic and the purist Mexican society, la bruja de rancho was a repository of accumulated ancestral knowledge. This knowledge was not institutionally recognized due to the systemic prejudice against woman, the machismo, and the lack of access to formal education that strongly marked those communities. Especially in little *ranchitos* in Mexico, the practices of the bruja de rancho also corresponded with the natural seasonal cycle, making the process of agricultural cultivation a very spiritual process. I come from a long line of farmers: my grandparents, Marcelino and Socorro, had a working farm.

The term bruja de rancho also describes my maternal grandmother Diana, a woman who, without need of credentials and degrees, put the benefits of her craft at the disposal of the people of our hometown. She was my greatest inspiration, mentor, and influence. My grandma made a living of doing readings, *amarres* (love and domination spells), and creating powerful amulets. By comparison, the only thing my Grandma Petra had on hand to work her magic were apples that had fallen to the ground. She had no time or resources for elaborate magic since she worked long hours at an orchard. They never hid their practices from us, but we were not obligated to follow them. However, they planted the seed in us, so when circumstances made it opportune or necessary, we knew what to do.

My learning was very casual, just like a baby would learn their mother's tongue. When you grow the way I did, there are no questions like, "what do those nails represent? And that ring? A tear? Those scissors? A horseshoe? A key? What about this seed? What does that eye hang on the wall for?" You just learn to understand some correspondence for each thing created in this universe. You learn another intrinsic language, understanding the magic everywhere. Their magic was very folkish, rudimentary, and practical, just like people in the Rancho are, but I got incredibly lucky that my abuela Diana married my grandpa, a knowledgeable brujo and a skilled tarot reader who was always studying magic.

I have to say that when I was young, I used to complicate my magic a lot. I wanted to make my grandfather proud of me. I even went so far as to say I would never do Brujeria de Rancho! But life itself put me in situations where I learned that even with extremely limited economic resources, lacking any purchasing power, Brujeria de Rancho was accessible for me. The purpose of this book is not to justify my path, to label it or satisfy my ego, but to give to the community the same tools, mechanics and knowledge that was given to me.

I am convinced that there is a complex confluence of events, energies, and circumstances that determines our predestined mission in life. The fact that you are reading this book right now is one of those magical confluences. Folk practices, witchcraft included, are not something typically learned in a formal school environment. Instead, these traditions are passed along orally and informally from one individual to another. Are you ready to start a tradition and work with your goals in the most Mexican of magical ways? What an honor to be the one who starts a long-lasting family tradition or to be the one who reconnects your whole family to it. Now is your time to accept, embrace, and make peace with it, and claim our ancestors' gifts. Each family has its own unique folklore; like a lot of Mexicans and Mexican-Americans, mine just happened to be magical. I'm pretty sure your family is as magical as mine, you may just need to start digging a little bit.

The purpose of this book is to help you connect or reconnect with Mexican magic. For some of you, this connection may trigger a sense of alienation, a feeling of not belonging. I want to tell you that whether you are in good standing with the Catholic church or not, whether you belong to a different religion, whether you consider yourself Mexican, half-Mexican, or not Mexican at all, this book and this legacy is for you. I hope to plant seeds in you of victory, love, joy, prosperity, luck, knowledge, creativity, connection, and belonging that will grow tall, and in turn plant other seeds of the same breed and continue this endless magical cycle. Do not forget that every act of magic operates like a seed and, like a rancher, cultivate an attitude of expectancy. Stay faithful.

Etymology: Brujeria, Hechicería, Brujeria de Rancho

All words are important, but some words matter more than others. Some have the power to change reality, the power to create, to heal, to harm, to destroy. Words can build up or tear apart. Words have weight. Words are magic. Because of this, I want to start saying that this book was dreamed and thought up in Spanish, which is my first language, but written and manifested into reality in English, my second language. One of Spanish's grammatical rules is that when the plural noun refers to a mixed group of genders, we use the masculine plural form for definite articles and adjectives. In other words, the rule is that in a group of mixed men and women, the masculine plural is used, even if there is only one man in a large group otherwise composed of women. (This grammatical rule is shared by many languages.) Thus, the word brujos can be used as plural for brujas, brujos, and all genders. When I use the words brujo or bruja, or a specific pronoun, I'm referring to people of every gender, including trans and nonbinary people, and celebrating all aspects of identity and expression across the spectrum. They are all included and celebrated in Brujeria de Rancho. This path is for each and every one of you.

It is necessary to discuss some of the terminology used in this book. The terms *hechicería* (sorcery) and *brujeria* (witchcraft) have been used interchangeably in Mexico, not only in major pre-Hispanic studies but also in published books and treatises by the Catholic church. A lot of times these studies, books, and treatises contradicted each other and themselves, causing confusion. To demonstrate how contradictory and confusing the use of these terms can be, one of most famous and important books of brujeria in Mexico is called *El Libro De San Cipriano, Tesoro Del Hechicero (The Book of Saint Cyprian: The Sorcerer's Treasure)*. The title—"The Sorcerer's Treasure"—suggests that it is a tome of hechicería, not of brujeria. As you can see, the words are often used interchangeably.

Brujeria is a broad term used by millions of people in the Spanish speaking world and is not limited to Mexicans or Mexican-Americans. Today in Mexico, people use the term "bruja" to refer to any person who practices any form of magic, including divination and astrology, even if they don't practice something conventional or traditionally Mexican. While many Mexican anthropologists have drawn a distinction between "witch" and "sorcerer or sorceress," the words continue to be used interchangeably among the population. Even among practitioners, these terms are often very fluid. I want to be clear that the word brujo or bruja does not necessarily carry the same connotations as in other Latin American countries. In Mexico, the word "brujo" has acquired a lot of political undertones, and usually means a person who is inconvenient to the establishment or system. I would say that these meanings vary from region to region, but to be completely honest, in thirty-seven years I have never met a practitioner of the craft in Mexico who puts themselves into a box with those meanings. Personally, I don't feel the necessity to pigeonhole myself. What matters is the work that we are doing and the help that we are providing to people in our communities. As practitioners, we are judged by our results. Our ability is not validated through titles or vanity labels.

The words *brujo* and *hechicero* have their own folk etymology and historical development according to a specific area but I would like you to understand some basic academic concepts that define these practices in Mexico. The main difference between brujeria and hechicería are that the methods employed. Hechicería's methods are more traditional and generally based on the close relationship and interaction that the hechicería has with their local environment. The main ingredients of rituals, spells, and concoctions are foraged from this environment, and the knowledge of the craft is mostly passed from person to person, generation to generation. Brujeria by contrast is more specific, ritualistic, and precise about planetary hours, astrology, planetary colors versus vibratory colors, and metals used for talismans. It is more ceremonial than hechicería.

In Mexico, brujeria is a practice that is contextualized in a historical period and specific area. It corresponds to both pre-Hispanic and colonial development. A pact with the devil (or demons) made with the intention of achieving a higher good that is otherwise obstructed is what gives the brujeria the heretical character in our folklore and what completely separates it from hechicería.

By contrast, hechicería's beginnings were very sexual. Many hechiceras were women confident in their sexuality who used magic to level up their sexual performance and to trap a man of a higher class. There is a distinct erotic touch to the stories of hechiceras in every file of the Mexican inquisition. Traditionally speaking, these women didn't want to hide. They wanted to be seen and admired and used a variety of plants for makeup in order to better themselves and their living conditions. We can't separate these goals and mechanics from the practice. Hechicería practices may or may not imply an association with the devil, demonic entities, and the use of malicious magic to carry out tasks without a pact or an exchange, only collaboration. A hechicero (sorcerer) today may or may not transgress upon religious beliefs to either rid people from evil intentions—or subject people to them.

In this book, I place folklore into context, providing a deeper understanding about what a Brujo de Rancho is in Mexico. Brujo de Rancho is a term used to refer to individuals who master combinations of brujeria, hechicería and *ensalmacion* (folk healing), folk psychology, and necromancy. It's wrong to reduce the practices of the Brujo de Rancho to a simple skill or two. I know that I am challenging the definitions placed, but Brujos de Rancho are not one-dimensional.

CHAPTER ONE

BRUJERIA DE RANCHO

*"Magic has always belonged to those who didn't have anything else
to fall back on except magic."*

—J. Allen Cross, author of American Brujeria

Since their earliest days, Mexican people have believed that their destiny was influenced by occult forces. The first civilizations in Mexico had their own beliefs on how to perform rituals; however, with the introduction and addition of various European and African rites, a new way of magic was born.

What is Brujeria de Rancho?

Brujeria de Rancho is an ancient practice, born, developed, and practiced mostly in rural areas of Mexico as a fusion of pre-Hispanic and colonial beliefs, where Catholicism and pre-Hispanic sorcery collided together and gave birth to this esoteric path. The practice of Brujeria de Rancho is a way to connect to our roots, our lore, our ancestors, and our traditional legion of spirits, both those who were already part of our land and those who happened as a result of colonialism, those folk spirits born from our fractured Mexico. Brujeria de Rancho is a perfect balance between Mexican brujeria, hechicería, ensalmería, and folk magic. This practice combines the sacred, the unhallowed, the sacrilegious, the heretical, and the macabre. Since Brujeria de Rancho is an ancient practice based on ancestral traditions, it is composed of very diverse praxes that have been brewing through the last six centuries.

La Brujeria de Rancho is the sorcery that I was taught. More than an institutionally recognized practice, it is an everyday occurrence, my lifestyle, my predecessors' lifestyle. It is cause and effect, a combination of pre-Hispanic and colonial influences, the response to terrible actions and the ensuing unfortunate chain of horrible events in Mexico. One example is how brujas de rancho began doing a lot of prosperity spells in 1982, following the devaluation of the peso when the ability to obtain foreign exchange weakened. My grandmother used to say that Brujeria de Rancho is like the revolution, something powerful that makes fear switch sides, something violent used to injure, defeat, or destroy, to tear down and overthrow, meant to uproot. Brujeria de Rancho can represent power; it is Saint Michael's sword to slay demons and conjures changes in our luck. But it can also be used to summon those same demons to be our allies and change our fate. To many, Brujeria de Rancho is devotion mixed with *café de la olla,* the comforting familiar blanket under which we hide to protect ourselves when the world is cold. All of these versions are completely true! This is what makes this form of magic so miraculous.

Mexico's social inequity is the mother that births all brujos and brujas de rancho. It is a parent who came to motherhood through undesirable situations, the one who has shown us her most cruel and toxic face. Our father is the culture of corruption, the weakness of Mexican state. La Brujeria de Rancho did not incubate in the minds of occultists, nor in the lodges of the privileged; la Brujeria de Rancho had its cradle where our people suffered, sprouted from the hands of "powerless people," *la gente del rancho,* or people from rural areas in Mexico, the excluded and the forgotten. Brujeria de Rancho was created out of the necessity of our people who were looking for a grip, a foothold, and who had no trust in the authorities, representatives, or the Church itself. Brujeria de Rancho is the vindication of popular anger, the embodiment of justice, the people's revenge, and the violent destruction of injustice. It is our response to impunity.

To further the parent metaphor, Brujeria de Rancho also takes on the role of guardianship. It endeavors to supply better living conditions where people have been unjustly abandoned by the State: such as health care, social welfare, a sense of security, and justice. As a brujos de rancho, we are not only expected but also required to do whatever needs to be done to protect, help, and empower our families and the members of our communities. We understand the responsibility that this entails, and that is the only "moral code" that we live and die by. These brujos are present mainly among poor peasants and workers; the unemployed and sick; those without social assistance; people who are disabled; the neglected elderly; housewives who struggle to support their children or who deal with abusive husbands or partners; undocumented immigrants and all of those who have had no other option than the Brujeria path.

A brujo de rancho is kind of a *sicario*—a spiritual hitman. Traditionally they are very discreet and ask only the most minimal, needed questions. Since the beginning of this practice, Las Brujas and Brujos de Rancho were strong and resilient people. They understood that a curse or hex is a means of seeking a redress of balance. It is the way that we address impunity and injustice, sometimes the only way available for us and our people, for those who have no other resources. This is a job not meant for the faint of heart; if you lack courage or have no sense of social justice, this practice is not for you. Brujeria de Rancho has been, is, and will always be a tool for rebellion; it has to do with equality, defiance, and a response to injustice and oppression.

It needs to be said that drawing a line between Catholicism and Mexican magic is useless for Brujeria de Rancho practitioners, the equivalent of trying to hold water in our hands and stretching them out in front of us. There is no point in drawing this line because it does not add or take away anything from this practice. As Brujos and Brujas de Rancho, our beliefs are not dictated by the Catholic church, or whatever may be their current posture about life choices such as abortion, marriage equality, or euthanasia. Brujeria de

Rancho practitioners condemn the atrocities and abuses perpetrated by the Catholic church and their clergyman not only in Mexico but also everywhere in the world. For Brujeria de Rancho practitioners, the church is a mean to an end. Brujos de Rancho are the biggest proof that Mexican faith resists and persists. When the institution in charge sought to contain, protect, and express that faith, their methods were shown to be far from social reality. We were the other alternatives that were sought. This is the reason why there is no traditional Brujeria Mexicana without the framework of Catholic beliefs: if you take either folk Catholicism or heresy out of the equation, or you add the church as an institution, then you are practicing something else.

But what do we mean when we talk about heresy? The word "heresy" derives from a Greek word meaning "choice." Mexican brujos believe in whatever we choose to believe, meaning that our beliefs exist outside of all forms of structure dictated by organized Catholicism. Traditional Mexican Brujos are guided by our own sense of right and wrong, dictated by our own interest and the interests of our community.

Brujeria de Rancho is our way to rescue what our ancestors left to us and use it to our favor. It was how our ancestors searched to achieve personal wellbeing, to escape the influence, dominion, and control of others. It is meant to be subversive, manipulative, disruptive and extremely raw. Brujeria was our ancestors' weapon, a force of spiritual coercion to help ourselves and others to meet our wants or needs. It is spiritual corruption conduct by those in power, typically involving bribery, pacts, alliances, sometimes with the goal to make other people do something that they do not really want to do, or give up things that they don't really want to give up. Brujeria Mexicana belongs to the wicked, the cunning, and those with no scruples, and unless you are in peace with that fact, you are not going to succeed. This practice was created by those experiencing extreme oppression who needed their wits and cunning to survive, and the practice to this day reflects that.

It is important for you to know that there is no uniform, solidified Mexican Brujeria or Hechicería practice. While a lot of Mexicans and Mexican

Americans do share similar practices, the idea that there is an only one right way, a solely Mexican authentic or traditional way to practice, is frankly ludicrous. Traditions are ways of responding to reality, to the environment, to the needs of the people. They are teachings adapted over and over again. Spiritual and magical practices are not pure uncontaminated intellectual enterprises, nor are they self-contained entities; they are influenced by a variety of interests, parts of a larger whole. In other words, we are all influenced by experience. Each tradition and practice in Mexican witchcraft is the product of a complex host of experiences collected over innumerable lifetimes. With this being said, I don't want you to think you can make it into whatever you feel like and turn it to something else that brujeria is not. The lived experiences that shaped these practices and traditions must be respected.

Brujeria and Hechicería Mexicana work with their primary two roots without cutting either, both pre-Hispanic and colonial, and faithfully resemble the goals and mechanics that our ancestors had for this practice. My advice to those who are interested in beginning their Mexican witchcraft journey is to cultivate a deep interest in both Mexican history and geography, and to read the books of other Mexican practitioners. This book is not meant to be the end of the road for you, a be-all and end-all compendium, but rather a small collection of the wisdom and practices gathered through many generations of my family. Many perspectives are necessary to create a full and beautiful picture of Mexican witchcraft traditions.

Likewise, many people would think that the benefits of the Mexican magic that I offer in this book are not within their reach, or that this type of magic should be accessible only to those born and raised into this tradition who inherited directly just like I did. This view does not take into consideration that this practice is a lifestyle. It is not just about magic, spells, and remedies; it is about beliefs and values passed down through so many generations by welcoming people who were always willing to share. This knowledge did not necessarily have to be passed from blood relative to blood relative, but rather to those who were willing to learn from their elders. This book is not intended to be a book of theory or a history book.

There are many books available if you want that. Rather, I want to help you to tap into different ways of Mexican magic, not just one. What you have in your hands right now is intended to be very folkish and rancho-like. You have my roots, my ancestors' practice. I encourage everyone reading this book to feel welcomed and included. I want to leave this clear for you, and everyone reading this book: To be able to ask for spirit help has not been, is not, and never will be a special prerogative of any religion, race, or ethnicity; it has always been, is, and always will be the greatest gift that our divine creator gave to us all.

This compendium is designed in a simple and economical form so that anyone can learn from it just like my ancestors did. We will work our magic in a very rudimentary way and make it as practical and easy as they did. Brujos de Rancho did not run to the botanica every time they wanted to get work done, or order materials online, or follow complicated recipes. Traditionally speaking, that is not what Mexican witchcraft is about. Brujeria de Rancho survives through the simplicity, the beauty, and the accessibility of simple kitchen magical ingredients, and the empowerment that this gives to the marginalized. It is craft paper, natural jute cord, burlap bags, grains, seeds, garlic, rue, body fluids, and multipurpose tools. This is not a trendy, aesthetically pleasing practice. It is no surprise that capitalist appropriation of these practices continues to rise, not only in the US but also in Mexico. The reclamation of this practice must come from embodied stories, not expensive brujeria products or decontextualized subscription boxes. Brujeria de Rancho is not practitioners claiming folk titles when they have done nothing for the people or specific region in Mexico they claim to represent except profiting, writing books devaluing the practice, and making brujeria something that it is not, inventing some new certification that you "must have" to become a brujo when these practices were passed orally and genuinely out of love.

Don't get me wrong. It can be crucial for practitioners to be paid for their spiritual services in the same manner that other professionals are. For example, this is how my grandma made her living. She charged for her services and was paid for the classes she gave. However, the ultimate goal must be to empower you, connect you with a true tradition, customs, and history, not make you dependent on a cycle of consumerism. If you want to be traditional you must decapitalize the practice, quit mass consumption, and give up the false "glamorous aesthetic" that does not belong to our Mexican magical traditions. To take ownership of this, your practice doesn't need my permission, my validation, or that of anyone else. Books, materials, mentors, and social media are only examples, resources. Mexican magic is not an exact science. I want you to know that both of my grandmothers, who were powerful brujas de rancho, had diverse ways of doing things.

Our house, especially our kitchen, is full of magic elements and ingredients. Most of the ingredients are ordinary and easily accessible, like sugar, salt, cinnamon, chiles, vinegar, chocolate, piloncillo, rice, pepper, and oil, among others. Isn't it incredible that things that have an everyday use hide magical power? In this book, you are going to get to know these ingredients and to learn how to use them. I want you to feel confident and remember that magic (I'm not just talking about Mexican magic) is in the knowledge you inherited, in your flesh and bones, the raw inner spiritual part of yourself. You carry this energy, strength, and resilience in your DNA, passed down from your ancestors. Even if you don't have Mexican heritage, you have this calling for a reason.

Some of the spells in this book call for a prayer candle of a specific color. If you cannot get a prayer candle, or cannot find one in the called for color, get a plain candle. The white ones can be used for everything. Or simply light the stove and visualize the spirit that you need to help you. If you do not have a gas stove or the money to pay your gas bill (I wish you had an idea of how many times that happened to me while I was in Mexico) simply bring the pain that still burns you inside, and channel it to accomplish your purpose. It may not be ideal, but in Brujeria de Rancho, you work with what you have. The first usage of prayer candles in Mexico was not documented until 1952, and our ancestors were working their magic long before that.

Please don't feel discouraged just because you may be going through some hard times. Mexican brujos have always found a way. Remember that we are seeds and our process continues even in uncertainty and darkness.

Your ancestors walk with you, as do mine right now, so do not be afraid of what is coming. You are not alone; they are guiding you. That is one of the reasons why you are reading this book right now.

Somos Los Hijos del Maíz: People of the Corn

The colloquial expression "We are the people of the corn" dates back to pre-Hispanic times, when the indigenous peoples and founders of pre-Hispanic empires saw corn as a sacred element of nature from which it is believed man was created. The title of this section is perhaps the best way to frame the nature of this type of magic. American readers may only be familiar with the phrase in reference to the 1984 horror movie *Children of the Corn* based on Stephen King's short story of the same name. Our understanding of this phrase predates that and has nothing to do with King's reflections on small town America. The feeling of being sons and daughters of corn is a deep reflection of our Mexican magic. Corn in Mesoamerican cultures represented, in philosophical terms, the fundamental axis of existence on Earth. Corn generates life. Corn is Mexico, the life force of the people.

There is a lot of alchemy and magic in agriculture, especially corn. Corn has long been a source of spiritual and material life. In Mexico, its dogma and liturgy are history and legend: it is tradition, and it is still alive.

The word "maize" (from the Spanish *maíz*) literally means "What sustains life," and comes from the Taíno words *mahisi* or *mahis*. The origin of the maize plant is unknown; wide diversification does not allow a single origin to be clearly defined, which is why today it is called a "multicentric" plant. Despite the multiple theories and various evidence, no wild species has yet been discovered that can be said with 100% certainty to represent the ancestral form from which cultivated maize originates. Modern evidence indicates that Euchlaena Mexicana is the closest known relative of maize, yet the full story of maize domestication and subsequent radiation remains so far unresolved, although historical evidence indicates that its origin is Mesoamerican.

For Mexicans, maize is not only a crop, but also a deep cultural symbol intrinsic to daily life. The shapes, sizes, and colors of the traditional maize varieties cultivated by Mexican people are a reflection of ourselves. Corn is extremely diverse: ears of corn can range in size from a couple of inches to a foot long, and it exists in colors including white, red, yellow, blue, violet, black, and pink, with some beautiful varieties even have an assortment of colors on one ear. Of the 220 existing breeds of corn in Latin America, sixty-four are native to Mexico.

Just like Mexican food, Mexican magic is very much like Mexicans themselves: rich, vibrant, extravagant, flavorful, and remarkably diverse. The sap of its indigenous origins runs through its veins, and these origins later gave birth to a continuous process, like the cross-breeding of corn. It began with the Spanish conquest and its culture, enhanced by African, Arab, and Jewish influences, and then nurtured itself through other contributions that arrived later through war, commerce, and other reasons from China, France, Ireland, Lebanon, Germany, and others. Primeval indigenous civilizations are determining factors in this magic and its root, but we have a vast national territory and numerous branches that enhances regional diversity.

When we discuss Mexican cuisine or Mexican magic, we are talking about a huge collective of varied culinary or magic traditions, full of richness and diversity. Puebla, Nuevo León, Veracruz, and Oaxaca are only a few examples of how different these folk traditions and influences could be. I am from Northeastern Mexico. My ways of experiencing and practicing magic highly reflect this particular area and the ways of the people there, the Natives who inhabited the area: the Alazapas, Guachiles, Rayados, Coahuiltecan tribes, the Tlaxcalan colonizers of Northern New Spain (today Mexico and south Texas), and the presence of *Anusim*, descendants of Jews from the Iberian Peninsula who were forcibly converted to Catholicism in the 14th and 15th centuries. Keep in mind that Monterrey, the city where I was born and raised, was settled by 695 Jewish families who escaped the Inquisition.

For Mexicans like me, those born and raised in Mexico and in many cases still living there, being Mexican is not about a race, ethnicity, the place where you were born, or a matter of ancestry; it is completely and one hundred percent about identity. To mention the best example of our favorite Mexican representatives, the first one would be Chavela Vargas (R.I.P.), a Costa Rican born Mexican singer who was especially known for her rendition and contribution to the genre of Mexican *rancheras* music. In my opinion, the wisest quote said by a Mexican was hers, said very casually during a famous TV show interview. The reporter asked her, "Why are you continuously calling yourself a Mexican?"

She responded to him, "Por que yo soy Mexicana," *because I am Mexican.* He replied to her, "But Chavela, you were born in Costa Rica." She just smiled back at him and proudly remarked: *Los Mexicanos nacemos donde se nos da la re chingada gana,* which translates, "Mexicans are born wherever the fuck we want!"

Mexicanity involves a collection of wounds, but also celebration and optimism without exclusions or regulations. It is tolerant, not divisive. Mexicanity implies pride, a sense of community and the belief of bridges over walls. Mexicanity is the philosophical, historical, psychological, artistic, spiritual, and cultural vision that was inherited and assimilated in Mexico over hundreds of years, and are proud of the richness of their own heterogeneity. We can't expect Mexican folk practices to be pure. That would reduce our practice to being a magical fiction book. Mexican magic is the reflection of its people: diverse, rich, and *mestiza.* In Latin America, *mestiza/mestizo* means a mixed race person or a person of mixed race ancestry, especially of Indigenous, African, and Spanish descent.

There is a difference in definitions between the mestizo identity that was adopted by the Mexican nation-state in 1825, which was an attempt to transcend ethnic differences and build a unified Mexico in a country that still to this day is suffering ravages from the previous Casta System. The Casta System was a system enforced by the Spanish Empire to classify various races and combinations thereof. Today, we as Mexicans embrace this mestizo identity without its previous systematic baggage. Mexicans and

Brujos de Ranchos today identifying themselves as mestizo do so celebrating our African heritage and its contributions to our culture and our magic. For Mexicans today, being mestizo means carrying together our idiosyncrasies, our world view, our faith, our food, our medicine, and our magic, ingredients from both the Western and Eastern hemispheres.

It should be noted that despite the historical Spanish obsession with "pure blood"—*limpieza de sangre,* the 15th century Spanish concept of someone whose ancestry was completely Christian, lacking Jewish or Muslim ancestors—those who conquered Mexico were not even remotely as "pure" as some wished to believe. Essentially, the Spain that conquered Mexico was already a mestizo empire, as it, too, had suffered invasions and vassalage, as well as Moorish and Jewish influences. No one with Iberian heritage exists today without some "Moorish" or North African and Middle Eastern heritage, including most Mexicans.

Denying what is Spanish is as serious a mistake as denying what is Indigenous and African, as well as the contribution of so many generously magical, and spiritual cultures and contributions who arrived later. A great example is the Espiritismo of the French Hippolyte Léon Denizard Rivail (Allan Kardec) that arrived in Mexico during the Second French intervention in Mexico, popularized during the Mexican Revolution. Being mestizo in 2022 is a Mexican manifesto, in which all ancestors and contributors fit into the larger picture. We have no right to exclude a single one, nor to disrespect any of the sacred elements of Mexican culture.

A Guide to Working with Spirits
in Brujeria de Rancho

"Through her, I learned that my spirit
shared in the spirit of all things."

—Rudolfo Anaya, *Bless Me, Ultima*

Our ancestors were certain that everything in the world had a spirit. As such, hundreds of these spirits were asked to intervene to generate good crops, bring rain, cure or cause diseases and misfortunes. At present, this thought is not much different. Things like disease and bad luck are still thought to be the effect of ill will, and harmful spirits are often sent either consciously or unconsciously by other people. These beliefs never cease to echo and influence our practice, although today it may be hidden under Catholic beliefs. These underlying beliefs have always been present since the time of the Aztec and Mayan era and perhaps even much further back.

Spirits in Brujeria de Rancho are divided into various classes. The Supreme or Creator spirit is the one that governs everything, and to him, all created things, both spiritual and material, are absolutely subject. From that Creator spirit, all of the other spirits were created, and each fulfills their special mission in the universe and all absolutely obey the Supreme Spirit. It is a general rule in Brujeria de Rancho to admit as a truth the existence of both good and evil spirits, and to acknowledge their antagonism towards each other, but to also recognize that all fulfill their missions in accordance with the laws of their creation.

Brujeria de Rancho is an animistic practice, which incorporates the belief that everything in the universe is ensouled (possesses a soul or spirit) including humans, animals, trees, seasons, natural places such as lakes, oceans, mountains, and caves but also objects. All forms and shapes are interrelated because we share the same life force, since the Creator Spirit breathed life into all things.

Brujeria de Rancho is a devotional practice, one based on passionate loyalty. Usually, when we are devoted to something, we spend significant time and energy focused on that person or thing. As brujos de rancho, we develop significant devotion and relationships with the spirits, saints, and ancestors we work with, as well as plants and other natural phenomena. We offer observances such as prayers, services, and offerings, among others. Most Brujeria de Rancho folk spirits are characters who for the most part had a life of martyrdom and manifested gifts of healing and protection for the most beaten sectors in Mexican society. These spirits may vary from one brujo de rancho to another due to geographic location and necessities. Not all of us work with the same spirits.

Rather than considering the following guidelines as rules, I want you to understand that they will help and protect you and at the same time allow your magic to have a better rhythm and a positive outcome.

Do not work with what you do not know.

I am talking about taking the responsibility of having a spirit in your house. Keep in mind that, like any being, a spirit will have individual characteristics and instincts, a need to be fed, and a way to influence moods and emotions in every single person in the household. Those influences and experiences are not the same with every single spirit that you may invoke, they are not cookie cutter. Every time you read a spell to contact a spirit, first research that spirit and get a feel for how they will work with you.

If you want to start creating your own spells, workings, and rituals with the correspondence tables I added at the end of this book, try to look for a spirit who has a lot in common with you, or with the purpose of your working. For example, do not ask Emiliano Zapata for something that is not a fair cause, because that is not going to work well. If you are looking to create a bond with a spirit, there are some tips that you could try before you work with them. Although there is no magic secret to instantly click with someone, there are a lot of things that you can do, such as looking into their patronage or researching their myths and legends. Read about their life story, their profession, and the things that are important for them, to see what resonates with you.

Here are some additional tips for establishing a connection with a spirit or saint in the Brujeria de Rancho tradition. Try to investigate if your family is *encomendados* (entrusted) to a particular saint or folk spirit. Sometimes it may happen that one of your great great grandmas did a lot of service and prayers for a specific saint—this act of selfless devotion will help you, too. When communicating with a spirit or folk saint, be open and share your hardships. There is a lot of comfort and magic that is found only by doing so. Do something kind for people under the patronage of a spirit or folk saint—it doesn't have to be a big gesture, small ones are enough. Remember to listen well; you are going to start receiving messages. When you do, respect and honor those messages. Remember that this is a two-way relationship, especially if a spirit lets you know in one way or another that they will not work with you.

Understand that this relationship, like any other, will take time to grow and become stronger.

Show gratitude—a thank you note, a wildflower, a gesture. Not all contact that you are going to have with this being will be friendly at the beginning. That is why I encourage you to get to know the spirit or folk saint you are contacting first. I had a case of someone who wanted to work with Pancho Villa, the Mexican Revolution general now venerated as a folk spirit. He thought that including tequila among his offerings was a good idea. However, Pancho Villa was a teetotaler—his only addiction was strawberry shakes, which he tried for the first time in El Paso, Texas. Pancho Villa many times decreed the "dry law" and believed that drunkenness only caused poverty and ignorance in the Mexican people. On numerous occasions, he shot at canteens to close them when they did not comply with said law. Imagine how badly that offering went.

Some spirits require more attention and time than others.
You should not be playing with them unless you are 1000% committed to that relationship. Not all spirits work in the same way, which is why it is important to try working with one at a time.

Have a clear understanding of what you are trying to accomplish.
If you do not know what you want, how can you expect the spirit will know? It is easier to put a plan into action once you know what you are trying to accomplice.

Mental Magical Design
Magic is planned, so we have handy ingredients, times, a list, days of the week, and correspondences. Even though Mexican folk magic does not really rely on specific days or times of the day, when something becomes an urgent matter, it is highly encouraged to work with correspondences. Check the tables at the back of this book for more information.

Opening of the Ritual
Our ancestors always asked permission. They were respectful of spirits and entities, not entitled. You need to connect with that spirit to ask if they want to work with you. They are not your employees, or your pets to train at will.

Faith
Do not forget that Mexican folk magic is a field in which it is necessary to learn to be confident, to trust in the spirit. This is not the type of magic you are going to accomplish through your higher self. In this type of magic, you pull spirit, you are pulled, or you meet in the middle. If you are not the trusting kind of person, or if you are a person who has developed trust issues from traumatic life experiences, this traditional magic may not be for you, or you may need to work on becoming more trusting before attempting it.

Take into account that the New Age term "lightworker" is totally different from what a Mexican folk magic practitioner would experience in the praxis of the same concept. In the New Age tradition, a lightworker is driven by their internal guidance and their higher self. For us in the Mexican folk tradition, the term lightworker is completely literal—we understand that this practice is not supposed to be a lot of heavy work. This work is, literally, light, involving praying with your rosary, lighting a candle, and talking to your spirits. We have left the heavy lifting to them.

For Brujeria de Rancho practitioners, it is as simple as trusting in the spirits we are working and building relationships with them. The life situations you are working to resolve may bring about the feelings of uncertainty and anxiety. With this type of magic, you cannot stress. Faith is the key. We have been training for these situations all our lives and we know if we trust our magic and the spirit, we will achieve the desired outcome. Do your work and let it go.

Do your work.

Spirits help the diligent. Your intentions need to be aligned with your actions. This motto emphasizes the importance of self-urgency. Magic helps only as much. You need to put in the effort. If you want to have a relationship, download a dating app. Same goes for that dream job; start filling out applications. As much as I would like, the magic that I offer you in this book does not work like a magic genie lamp.

Balance

This guidance is coming from a long line of brujas de rancho. They worked the soil and were very deeply connected to the agricultural ways, so I want you to take this advice with the sowing the land approach because it is written 100 percent in that context.

Balance must not only be present in the elements to be used in your spell, but it must also be present in what we give and intend to take. As Brujeria de Rancho practitioners, we depend on the help of the spirit, so we can manifest what we want or need on the physical plane. In general, the exchange must be reciprocal. Whoever receives what is needed or wanted must in turn give back to the spirit.

Compensation is achieved only by giving back. The first balance disorder starts there, where one tries to reap fruit where he has not sown! Give *ofrendas* (offerings) in gratitude or devotion, or as a present or gift that is dedicated to the spirits or the saints to implore their help and to fulfill a vow or obligation.

Engage
I know I said that this is light work, but for no reason should it be taken lightly. Turn off your phone, turn off that TV, engage in your prayers, and spend quality time with the spirit. Interruptions are very discouraging when we are doing this type of work.

Be smart
This is a kind of practice that you are going to perform in your house. Be clean, be sanitary in both the physical and the spiritual; you have a visitor, an incredibly special one.

Keep in mind that if you plan to perform spells or rituals in other people's presence, you need to make sure these people have the same interests, or that those interests align with yours, otherwise this will not work in your favor.

Be honest
People who do magic must be extremely honest in their personal life and their opinions, without any fear of what other people may think or say, without fear of losing followers or fear of upsetting other magic practitioners with some uncomfortable truths—or at least, what is it true for them. Nobody owns the absolute truth, but we sure own our own, whatever it may be.

A bag of herbs, a candle, a spell—these acquire the power of whatever I want them to acquire because I say they will, but most importantly because

I am a woman of my word, a woman who always keep true to my truth and intentions.

For your word to acquire that strength, you must deeply and absolutely identify yourself with the truth. That principle must resonate with your life all the time. If I habitually lie, especially to myself, do not keep my promises, do not honor my word and my truth, and do not live my life accordingly with my truth, how can I expect my words to have the powerful strength to perform magic? You need to honor your pacts, your agreements, and your offerings.

Do not forget about the Divine Providence!

Divine Providence is God's intervention in the universe. It is the action of God and the resources that he gives to human beings so that they can subsist and develop; that includes this kind of magic. In other words, Divine Providence speaks to the superiority of God and the need that human beings have for His existence so that He can provide them with the necessary tools to lead a full life.

To be a recipient of Divine Providence, you must be a giver as well. Every time you ask for Divine Providence for yourself, ask for other people's providence too. This is the common denominator in every single Mexican folk magic practice: my ancestors were community people, and they cared about the community and its people. When they took, they gave in return.

Chapter Two

THE BRUJA'S KITCHEN

The kitchen is where we deal with the elements of the universe. It is where we come to understand our past and ourselves. Cooking is one of the strongest ceremonies for life. When recipes are put together, the kitchen is a chemical laboratory involving air, fire, water, and the earth.

—Laura Esquivel, *Like Water for Chocolate*

Many people find comfort and connection in making a permanent space in their home where they can find themselves at peace and are at ease with themselves and the spirit. This does not have to be fancy, just clean, safe, and practical. The kitchen is a great choice for many reasons. A well-appointed kitchen has running water, fire, and most of the things you are going to need to work this magic. The magical actions of our ancestors took place mostly in their kitchens, the place where everything traditional, magical, and worth passing on to the next generation begins. Since pre-Hispanic times, there has been nothing more precious than the kitchen. My abuela and my great grandma had their space in a corner in their kitchen, so do I. I keep that space always tidy, with water, a candle, my scissors, and spirit. Everything else is extra.

There is a historic association between the kitchen and witchcraft. Many ancient gods and goddesses are related to the kitchen and food in some way. Chantico is the Aztec goddess of hearth fires and precious things. Her name means "in the home." She is a force for women's magical arts, a domestic deity who lives in your fire and keeps your home safe and cozy. Aztecs prayed to Chantico to bestow wealth and stability upon their homes. According to Bernardino de Sahagún, the Aztecs came to think of her as a military deity, a goddess of war and the Protectress of their empire, since it was reported by the Spanish that the Emperor Moctezuma Xocoyotzin II did use a yellow effigy, with a removable leg is of the Aztec goddess as a tool to curse the land, obstructing the advance of Hernán Cortés.

It was on Chantico's day, the ninth day of the eighteenth trecena on the Aztec calendar, that witches turned into various animals and exercised their greatest power. *Mometzcopinqui* witches leave their legs with Chantico, represented by the stove bonfire that keeps their legs warm and protected. Mometzcopinqui are women born on the date of Ce-Ehecatl, which means "One-wind" or "One-rain." Women born on this date are said to develop certain supernatural abilities, including the ability to fly by removing their human legs. They were some of the most feared witches among the Aztecs.

Setting up a magic space can be as simple or as complicated (and expensive) as you want it to be. It's okay to start simple. You can have your contemplation altar or shrine somewhere else in your house while you do your workings in the kitchen. First and foremost, you must have a surface to do your workings on. Don't be a perfectionist about this—it doesn't have to be 100% perfect right from the start, just enough to set up on. You can always move it later on.

Here is a quick list of must haves for your kitchen workspace:

Barro (clay) plates and bowls: The cauldron of a bruja de rancho is made of clay. Clay is the representation of all the elements gathered together: earth and water are combined into mud kissed by the fire, dried in the sun helped by the air. Clay is the earth and it is our ancestors, because clay represents the entire universe and symbolically represents man. Barro, which literally means "mud" but generally means "clay," has been used in Mexico for generations, and can be found in almost every Mexican kitchen. It is a tradition passed down since pre-Hispanic times. In this practice, it is recommended that you stand your candles in this specific material as there is nothing more sacred to do spell work, or to contain it, than clay.

Cantarito Mexicano: a handmade pear-shaped jug made from pottery clay. Cantaritos have been used in various forms of Mexican folk music (Son Mexicano) and traditional dances and ceremonies as a percussion instrument.

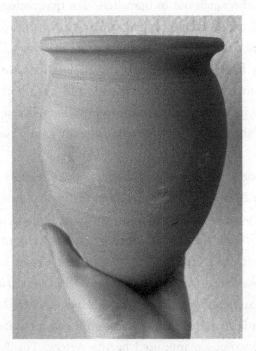

Jícara: A jícara is a vessel made with the peel of the fruit of the jícara tree. It is a tree native to Mexico. The gourd is associated with water, and its concavity can also be related to the springs that are under the hills.

Molcajete: The molcajete is a kind of traditional Mesoamerican mortar mostly used in Mexico. It is made of volcanic stone carved in a concave shape, which provides the ideal grinding surface for herbs, seeds, and other things you need to pulverize. (If you already have a mortar and pestle, you can use that instead.)

Grains, Herbs, and Seeds

"Tradition is not the worship of ashes, but the preservation of fire."

—Gustav Mahler

My grandmother used to say, "You can get the witch out of the ranch, but you can't get the ranch out of the witch." For that reason, my focus is not on herbs that are used in a particular place in Mexico or only where my ancestors were from. Rather, I encourage you to work with what you most likely already have in your kitchen, ingredients that are easily accessible in your supermarket or that your friends and neighbors have, if you are not currently in a financial position to buy them. These are the ingredients that our abuelas on the rancho had already handy every time they did "their thing."

Brujeria de Rancho is a very discrete and accessible practice. Do not expect to see New Age ingredients here. In this practice, if you don't tell the people in your household that you are doing brujeria, most likely they'll have no idea. This is the old-fashioned way to do Mexican magic.

If you want to start studying about herbs, seeds, and plants, I recommend researching *Libellus de Medicinalibus Indorum Herbis* (Códice De la Cruz-Badiano), and *The De la Cruz-Badiano Aztec Herbal of 1552* (Dover 2000), which is an Aztec herbal manuscript that describes the medicinal properties of various plants used by the Aztecs. The Badiano Codex is considered the oldest written text of medicine in America. This book is of great importance because it shows the work of our Indigenous people in medical matters, all based on the observation and use of natural elements, and most importantly it. The Badianus Codex, like the Florentine Codex, contains traces of humoral theory (the hot-cold polarity), the predominant western medical ideology of the era. Most brujas de rancho work with these two types of nature, which are part of the condition of multiple phenomena, like foods, colors, remedies, diseases, ailments. For example, hot represents masculinity, while cold is associated with the feminine. The days of the week also have different natures; Tuesdays and Fridays are hot days, for example. In rancho agriculture, chemical fertilizers are cold, while manure is hot.

Classifying diseases as hot or cold makes a lot of sense in our view, since it affects whether the remedy or the malediction should be hot or cold. The effect of opposites is generally used. That is, if the person has acquired a hot disease, then the remedy will be cold. This concept will help you understand not only why I say that Mexican Brujeria and our magic comes from several roots, but also how to design your hexes, curses, or remedies. Although it is generally agreed that the same diseases are not hot or cold for all cultures, there is usually a certain consensus.

Talk to Your Herbs and Seeds

Many of us are immigrants, or the descendants of immigrants. When you emigrate, the connection with your ancestors and the spirit of your land emigrates with you to the country where you now reside. I know for a fact that the language and tools we use have such strong and deep roots to the land that they either die or mutate when we emigrate. Regardless of where la bruja emigrate, they will always use their craft. We are empowered by knowing we are the bridge between the world of the living and the spirits, the ones that connect our ancestors to our descendants. The connection with the spirits and with your ancestors will always be there. Although connection to the land is crucial, especially when we talk about working with plants, roots, and seeds, do not fall into the mistake of believing that your relationship with your land is going to be the same as the one your ancestors had with theirs. This especially applies to plants that grow in specific areas.

It's important for you to take lessons from the past, but never sacrifice the future for the sake of continuity. We gauge decisions based on the present, and we understand that tradition is about both the mechanics and relationship with the spirit. Sometimes we can forget one of the most basic and important principles of the practice of plant-based witchcraft: the relationship to the land and the accessibility of the plant. The use of herbs, seeds, and grains is emergent, relational, practical, and dynamic. Their standardization is harmful because it becomes extractive, capitalistic, and removed from context. Do I encourage you to learn about plants and seeds such as ololiuhqui, peyote, tlapatl, mixitl, nanacatl, tochtetepon, toloache/datura, and many others used by natives in Mexico? Yes! Do I recommend taking them out of their habitat and environment, contributing to deforestation of sacred plants and seeds by trying to get them shipped to you to wherever you are? Absolutely not! That would be very irresponsible advice from my side. Understand that it's not enough to buy those ingredients; you need to have a connection and a relationship with their spirit for them to work.

I want to teach you the same way I was taught. The same mechanics, same principles, same Mexican magic, with ingredients that our people have been using for centuries: the ones in your body, in your pantry, the ones you are already familiar with, to which you have a connection already. To do otherwise, I would be leading you to a little to no results. It is a shame seeing brujas with a huge fear of using one plant instead of another, making unnecessary stops with their magic. I am not going to contribute to this madness because Mexican magic has nothing to do with this. Stop complicating your magic!

The first step is connecting with the spirit of your land. Many authors ignore where you physically are and the ancestral power of your local plants. At this moment, you could be contributing to the over consumption of *cocolmeca* or *Palma de todos los Santos* and ignoring the power of what is growing in your backyard or what you already have in your pantry.

Do you want to feel more confident replacing a plant? The breath of life is used in Mexican herbalism to awaken herbs with a specific intention, especially when you need to exchange one for another. It is as simple as inhaling deeply while envisioning how the energy of your creator is already in you. Exhale on the herbs, transferring that energy of life and letting the plants know their purpose. Wake them up and praise them. Praise is a form of prayer that recognizes the power of something or someone. Praise is a great weapon for spiritual warfare. When we praise something or someone, we are placing a great value on them. We are communicating to them what they are, what they have done, and what they can do for us. It helps us focus on the character and the attributes of a spirit. Our elders used to praise the power of herbs even before harvesting.

Talk to your herbs, explain what you are about to do, whether you are about to use the herb in a spell work, in a cleansing, or as a tea. Explain your need—why you are doing this and for whom. Don't forget to give thanks to the plant. State your faith that it will help you achieve your desire.

You can create your own prayers to awaken your herbs and imbue them with intentions. Here are examples of the two of the most popular folk prayers. It is believed that these prayers originated in the 16th century. Speak them with intention and awaken your herbs.

Powerful Rue

> *Blessed rue, powerful miraculous rue, that on Mount Calvary for the tears of Maria Magdalena you shed tears for me, give me luck, bring me prosperity, in the same way I ask blessed rue to bring me good business, to bring me happiness and bliss, to my body and soul. Amen.*

Blessed Rosemary

> *Blessed rosemary, lucky rosemary, beautiful rosemary, you were consecrated to God, you were born, you were sown, and with many goods you came accompanied. Blessed rosemary, flowering bush that grows free in the field, by the virtue that God has given you, transmutes all the bad into good, change my sorrows for joy, my poverty for riches, and my loneliness for love. Beautiful rosemary that attracts wealth, your beautiful flower brings me good health. Holy rosemary, blessed rosemary, rare is the sore that you cannot heal. Whoever touches you gets blessed the same day.*

Blessed rosemary that is in my house, protect my space and my possessions when I'm not there. Holy rosemary, blessed rosemary, make the bad go away and the good come my way. Amen.

Grains and Seeds in Brujeria de Rancho

It is no surprise that from the earliest times, seed planting was accompanied by a variety of rituals and magic. For our ancestors, bones and intentions were also considered to be seeds. A seed is a mystery, hope, heritage. prolific creativity, life and death, transformation, power, both nothing and everything. As we all know, there are various kinds of seeds. There are seeds that end up bearing fruit and there are seeds that spread bad weeds. Every seed has their correspondences, their associations, their folklore.

Protection Against Psychic Attacks and Witchcraft

You will need:

> *One red ribbon*
> *One alum stone*
> *Three corn seeds*
> *One corn husk leaf*

On a Tuesday, grab a medium size alum stone and the three corn seeds with your left hand and pray *the Magnificat* (if you are unfamiliar, you can find this prayer on the Internet). Wrap the alum stone and corn seeds with the husk leaf, making a little charm bag, and tie it with the red ribbon. Place it close to your pillow. In places with a lot of humidity, the corn will go bad, so replace it with new corn seeds whenever you think it is needed.

Rapid Money Spell with Yellow Corn

You will need:

> *Three $1 bills*
> *A Mexican clay bowl*
> *Seven yellow corn seeds*

A gold candle
White handkerchief

On a Sunday, place the three $1 bills and the corn seeds in the clay bowl. Light a gold candle and place it to the right of the bowl. Repeat the following three times:

> *By the divine providence, money comes easily to me and is multiplied three times each time I spend it and I receive it, in the name of the Father, the Son, and the Holy Ghost. Amen.*

Let the candle burn. When it is consumed, place the three $1 bills and the corn seeds in the white handkerchief. Leave it in a safe place in your house, preferably where you keep your money or your wallet.

Popcorn to Call Money and Abundance in Times of Need

Before the 16th century, popcorn, which the Aztec called *momochtli*, was already an integral part of Aztec ceremonies. It's common now for abuelas to place popcorn in clay bowls around the house to call abundance and prosperity. Every bowl should also contain one coin. If you have four people living in your house, place four bowls, and put a coin in every one of them. Say this prayer every time you are placing a bowl of popcorn in your house:

> *Corn's Divine Spirit, send your strength and protection from the deep. May the rays of the sun illuminate my path. Be my force in the hours of darkness. Loving creator of mankind, bless me with a rest that comforts me and the protection of my ancestors, be the blessing of my effort, the truce in hard work. Come Spirit Creator of life and bless me with an excellent harvest and the union of my family. You who are the nucleus, the seed, the wealth, my projects that germinate the flesh of my father, the blood of my mother, the bones of my children, of all our ancestors and those who will come through us. Amen.*

Chocolate

Chocolate has the powers to arouse emotions, change moods, and transfer us to an irresistible neurosensory experience. The cacao plant's origin is well established in South America, as is its consumption in the Olmec and Maya regions. The Aztec culture incorporates it into its oral tradition narratives that explain the origin of their mythology.

Chocolate has many wonderful stories attached to it, and those that relate to traditional Mexican witchcraft should not be missed. Since pre-Hispanic times, chocolate was served in marriage ceremonies and used in medicine and in rituals. Hot cocoa was not only the main object of paranoia among the Spaniards, but also an addiction and a sinful pleasure. Men associated chocolate with fear of losing their virility by being "bewitched" by their women and sexually dominated by them. Emperor Moctezuma, by comparison, drank chocolate before visiting his wives. And when chocolate was imported to Europe in the 17th century, it was considered that "decent women" should not taste it.

The vast majority of records in the files of the Mexican Inquisition list chocolate as one of the most used ingredients for brujeria. You can use Mexican chocolate tablets or organic cacao powder for spells and to dress your candles. With its aphrodisiac qualities, chocolate can bring the wooed to their knees and boost the libidos of any person with its magical aphrodisiac properties.

Chocolate to Invoke Sexual Desire

Whether you want to excite lust in an existing partner or cause someone new to lust after you, this is the right spell for you.

You will need:

An image of Anima Sola
One white candle
Two red figure candles
Organic cocoa powder

A wooden toothpick
Patchouli oil
Matches
Barro plate
Your pubic hair

On a Friday, begin by praying three Hail Marys to the Anima Sola. Light a white candle for her. Regarding your red figure candles, make sure to select one candle that represents you and the other to represent your intended. For example, if both you and your intended identify as women, select two female figure candles; if you are a woman and your intended a man, select one female and one male figure candle. (For those who identify as nonbinary, there are currently figure candles intended to represent you, as well!) Rub the two figure candles with the patchouli oil while focusing on the person in whom you want to excite lust. Grab the toothpick and write both the name of this person and your own name (or the name of the person you are doing the spell for). After that, dress both candles with cocoa. Rub your pubic hair only on the candle that represents your target.

Light your target's candle, but not yours. (You need your target's head to be hot, figuratively, but yours should remain cool.) Have the burning candle facing the unlit one as you repeat the following, filling in the parts in parentheses with your target's information:

> *Oh, Anima Sola, I stand in front of you to desperately request that you make (person's name) to want my body, my sex, and feel lust every time (their pronouns) sees me or hears my name. You, who knows the desires of my heart and my desperation to be with (person's name) sow in (person's name) the need to come to my side. You, who know how to inflict carnal desires, lust, and obsession. May (person's name) attraction be multiplied towards me and make (their pronouns) despair until (their pronouns) come like a dog in heat looking for me, to passionately make love to me until I get tired of it. Amen.*

Save the figure candle that represents you. Melt it down and combine it with the residual wax from the candle that represented your intended. Combine this wax with cacao butter and patchouli and create a new candle of the mixture. Burn this candle during one of those sexual encounters. You will have the best sex of your life.

Sweetenings with Piloncillo

Piloncillo or *chancaca* comes from the Nahuatl *chiancaca*, which means "brown sugar." It is prepared from the undistilled juice of the sugar cane, a raw form of pure cane sugar that is commonly used in Mexican cooking (and also in love magic potions and spells) since 1519, the time of the conquest of Mexico by the Spanish, when the cultivation of sugar cane was introduced. Piloncillo was the main source of sweetener for peasants and rural dwellers, and it is one of the principal ingredients used in Brujeria de Rancho. So, how do you use it? The piloncillo blocks look almost like gold ingots, and are made by reducing raw cane sugar juice into a thick syrup and then pressing it into dense bricks or cones. Piloncillo is available in many supermarkets. Use it for *endulzamientos* (see below), amarres, amulets, attractions, and offerings.

Unless otherwise instructed, don't dress your candles with piloncillo; since it is full of sugar, it will quickly caramelize. In spells that do call for you to dress a candle with piloncillo, please note that it requires only a very tiny amount. Using too much will prevent your candle from burning properly.

Endulzamiento: Sweetening

An endulzamiento or sweetening is a spell used when a relationship, be it familial, work, friendship, or romantic, is in crisis or going through tensions and disputes. The purpose of a sweetening is to resolve grievances. There must always be a relationship between the subjects; you can't perform a sweetening for people who don't already have some type of relationship. Sweetenings are used to "sweeten" a person's positive feelings and keep negative ones away. This transformation means that everything that can be extracted from this type of spell is very positive. Sweetening calms the waters, brings peace, love, and calm, as it makes each person predisposed to bring out the sweetest and most peaceful, understanding, and cooperative side of themselves, thus avoiding tensions.

Sweeteners can be seen as a love spell or as a soothing spell. They are traditionally more benign than amarres, which are love and domination spells. It is sometimes recommended that you try a sweetening before an amarre, as this kind of spell work is often enough to achieve good results; however, it all depends on the people and the circumstances. Regarding relationships with a partner, sweetening allows a person to return feelings of affection or good disposition back toward the other person, and grants the return of happiness where there was distance, coldness, or even aggression. If your goal is to save a relationship, a sweetening is something I would recommend.

You will need:

A glass jar with a lid
One piloncillo cone (eight ounces)
Two cups of water
A candle (check the color correspondence table in the back
  of this book to tailor it for your relationship)
A pen
Photo of the person to sweeten
Optionally, for a spiced version, add two cinnamon sticks and one
  whole clove. This variation is specifically for love matters.

Combine the piloncillo in a saucepan with the water and spices. Simmer over low heat until the piloncillo is fully melted, then increase the heat and bring to a boil. Keep boiling over medium-low heat, stirring frequently, until the syrup is thick enough to coat a spoon, about 10-15 minutes. Keep an eye on it while it cooks, as piloncillo syrup is prone to spilling over very quickly. Take it off the heat.

When the syrup is finished, take the picture of the sweetening target and write your desires on the back of it: that this person becomes more affectioned, obtains serenity, that barriers between you are eliminated and you become closer again, that a hot temperament is lowered. Be specific. Anything you think would bring you closer to and renew good terms with this person, write it down. Write your own name at the end.

Put the picture in the jar and pour the piloncillo syrup over it. Fill the jar completely with the syrup. Close the jar and place the candle on top of the lid. You must put it into *velacion* to give light to your work. In brujeria terms, "velacion" means to put something close to a candle light for the amount of time required for your working. Use a pink candle for a love relationship, white to harmonize family matters, blue for teachers and coworkers. It is best to do this on Friday for love, Wednesday for communication, work, or school-related relationships), or on Sunday when everything shines and you have the power of the sun, depending on what kind of relationship you are looking to sweeten.

If you cannot find piloncillo, other commonly used ingredients to perform a sweetening are corn syrup, honey, and *grageas* (sugar sprinkles).

To Tame and Control

Misogyny and machismo are a dangerous threat for Mexican women. Indigenous women, trans women, and pregnant women are especially targeted. Domestic violence, violence perpetrated by partners, violence that is the result of conflicts with neighbors, vendettas, and harassment are frequent dangers. The cruelty, brutality, and sadism present in this violence against women is concerning, as is the level of impunity that allows criminals to perpetrate these heinous crimes. This is nothing new. It is engrained in Mexican culture, normalized to the point where the rise of gender violence songs has become a worrying success.

Music is the reflection of the issues we face as a society. When the song "Hay Que Pegarle a la Mujer (You Have to Hit the Woman)" premiered in 1987, machismo was a cultural attitude on a large scale in the North. The

Mexico of the '80s and '90s proved propitious for this song, allowing it to be recorded and accepted without facing criticism for its shocking and violent lyrics. In a femicidal country like Mexico, where ten women are murdered on average daily for the simple fact of being women, the issue becomes more relevant.

The following ritual is appropriate when you want to calm and control a violent or aggressive person. It is for domination over someone, allowing you to be in control of them and granting you the power to defeat them. This spell is to establish your position of power and control over a lover, partner, spouse, and even grown-up children. If things escalate with a violent or controlling partner, leave and seek help. Our grandmothers might not have had that option, but we do.

You will need:

A wide mouth glass jar, such as a mason jar or a baby food jar
Balsamo tranquilo (calm balm oil, available at botanicas)
One cordero manso candle or a white candle
Baby blue ribbon
Black ink or a black pen
A photo of the person you want to calm
Corn syrup
Datura (Datura is a poisonous plant. If it is not avail-
* able locally or you prefer not to use it, use valerian.)*

Place the calm balm oil in a wide-mouth jar. (If you can't find calm balm, a good substitute is Passiflora tea. Passiflora is known as a calming plant in Mexico; although the plant can't be grown for consumption in the US, you can obtain herbal teas from various tea companies.) Take the picture and write on it the following prayer:

> *Through the meek little lamb, I conjure you (name of the person you want to tame) in the name of Jesus, Mary, and Joseph, and with these same words I conjure you again to come to me as a meek lamb full of love and attention towards me. O creature of God!*

Meek, meek as the meek lamb. Tranquil and quiet you are. You won't
scream. You will not shout. You are at peace with me and with your-
self. Gentle, gentle, kind, kind, calm, calm, you'll finally settle down.
You won't be upset anymore, not even at war, you will walk with a
happy face. Meek, like a meek lamb. Meek, like a meek lamb, you
(name of the person to tame) will finally be. So be it and so it is.

Once you have done this, pour the corn syrup over the photo. Roll it up and tie it with the ribbon and place it in the jar with the calm balm, then add the datura or valerian. Close the jar. Put the jar in velacion next to the cordero manso or baby blue candle. As you do this, envision the person in question becoming calm and doing whatever it is you want them to do. When the candle has been consumed, the jar must be buried without ever seeing the sunlight.

Chile

Chile has been the fundamental ingredient since pre-Hispanic Mexico. It characterizes the national cuisine and much of our identity and our magic. The chile had a very important role among the Aztecs, who used it as an element of payment of tribute to the authorities. The chile deity is the sister of Tlaloc and Chicomecóatl. Her name is Tlatlauhqui-cihuatl-ichilzintli, which means "Respectable lady of the red chile."

In Mexico, chile peppers are used and recognized as an effective tool against the Evil Eye, witchcraft, bad airs, and evil in general. They are used for protections, banishments, and cleansing due to their spiciness, red color, and shape. People who fear someone putting brujeria on their food usually eat it with a lot of chilies, since it is believed to prevent the absorption of the evil. To this day we light charcoal in rooms or enclosed places and burn handfuls of chilies as a method of healing, cleansing, and purification. Chile smoke has the power to remove discomfort in the respiratory tract and clear congestion as well. In brujeria matters, chilies are used to cause and create discomfort and heat.

Chile Serrano: Helps to remove negative vibrations, stagnation, black magic spells. Used to both remove and cause hexes.

Chile de Arbol: Favorable for cleaning physical spaces such as home or businesses; heat and speed up situations.

Chile Pasilla: Helps to remove the Evil Eye, low vibration beings, negative thoughts, and bad entities.

Chile Cascabel: binding and banishing.

Chile Guajillo: Opens roads. The seed serves for the good resolution of legal issues, contracts, and legal stationery.

Chile Piquin/chiltepin: Helps with banishing and exorcisms.

Chile Ancho: sexual, love, lust endeavors , black magic, and cleansing.

Chile Habanero: retreat, exile, lust.

Chile Magic

To cleanse yourself and harm an enemy: Tie seven dried chilies (any kind you have) together with a red string and pass them seven times over your body, from your head to your feet. Afterwards, sprinkle a splash of alcohol over the chile bundle and burn it by throwing a lit match on it. (Always be aware of fire safety!) Once it has burned all the way, sweep the ashes and throw them in your worst enemy's house.

To keep your partner from straying: Buy two large Pasilla chiles and arrange them in the form of a cross. Tie them together with a red ribbon. Place that chile-cross along with a Santa Elena medal or prayer card under the mattress where you sleep with your significant other, and stop worrying. Your significant other won't be able to leave that bed to sleep with anyone else.

To attract a particular lover: Cut open a chile Mulato, a dried version of a fresh poblano that tastes somewhat like chocolate or licorice, with undertones of cherry and tobacco. Place the picture of the person you would like to have sex with you inside the chile, along with a chunk of piloncillo and cinnamon. Wrap the chile within a piece of your worn but unwashed underwear and bury it in the ground or in a pot with a plant on top to hide it.

To Spiritually Clean Your House

You will need:

Ajo macho (male garlic)
Mexican clay bowl
Two Serrano chiles
Salt

On the first day of the month, or whenever you feel you need to remove bad luck or illness from your house, pour some salt in a clay bowl and on top of it add two chiles in the shape of a cross. Add the ajo macho at the foot of the cross. Leave them there until the chiles wither and then replace them, along with the salt and the male garlic, with new ones.

To Drive Away Someone Who Is Harming Your Relationship

This spell will help you to drive away someone who does not understand limits and is a constant annoyance and hindrance to your relationship. It will help you to remove this person from your relationship. The goddess Tlazolteotl both inspired carnal acts and absolved them and created and healed disease (usually sexually transmitted). She is the Aztec presiding goddess of witches. It was said that Tlazolteotl would afflict people with disease if they indulged themselves in forbidden love, so if you want to protect your significant other and your relationship, follow this spell.

You will need:

A photograph of the meddling person (nowadays it is quite easy
    to print a photograph taken from social media)
A white candle
A broom
Chile ancho powder

Place the picture of this person on the floor and sprinkle chile ancho powder on top of the picture. Start sweeping toward the door while you repeat the following statement:

Powerful broom of Tlazolteotl, sweep (name of the person),
my significant other's sins away, and place them in the trash, which
is where they belong, and sweep and clean the relationship of (your
name and your significant other's name, or the name of the couple
you are doing this spell for) of all envy, curses, and meddling of the
enemy. Amen.

Once outside of your house, pick up the photo with a dustpan and place it in a black trash bag. Throw it away in a trash can far away from your house.

Apples

Apples have been used for centuries in magic and rituals and have been the center of many mythological stories and Bible tales. Apples feature heavily in love magic. A sweet and often red fruit, apples are perfect for building a crush or new relationship into a strong loving relationship full of passion and lust. But make no mistake, apples are also very helpful in getting rid of our enemies because their seeds contain cyanide.

The journey of apples to Mexico was part of the long relationship between apples and humans, during the course of which this fruit has been spread to nearly every part of the world. With the exception of the wild sour crab apple, apples are not indigenous to North America, their cultivation originated in the mountainous region of the Middle East. Apples arrived in Mexico when the Spanish brought them; they were used it to make cider, vinegar, and wine. My great grandparents were orchard workers in Arteaga, Pueblo Magico in Coahuila, which is called the "Mexican Swiss Alps." Arteaga is famous for its red and golden apples, so everything related to "forbidden fruit" guarantees quality, including their magic. My Grandma Petra loved to work her magic with apples. She had so many stories around them that would be impossible for me to write them all, but these were her favorite apple spells.

Ven a Mi: Come to Me Trabajo

To attract love into your life, find a new lover, or give your current relationship a boost when your significant other seems distant and the relationship is cooling off. This spell can also be used to get back with your ex, as well as attract new potential partners.

You will need:

One Ven a Mi, pink or red candle
Honey
A red apple
A red ribbon
Cinnamon powder
Piloncillo
White paper
A pen with red ink
A barro plate
A knife

On a Friday, dress a candle with cinnamon and a tiny amount of piloncillo. (As a note, piloncillo tends to caramelize.) Clearly envision the person you would like to attract as you de-core the apple. Write on the paper with your red ink pen the characteristics and features of the person you would like to attract or the name of your target. When you are finished, put a layer of honey, piloncillo, and cinnamon on top of the paper. Put the paper inside the cored apple and glue everything together with the honey. Tie the apple with the red ribbon, making sure that it will not open by making three strong knots.

Say the following prayer:

> *Come to me, burning and passionate love, come to me. At this holy moment, I dominate your being and your thoughts, subject your mind through the influence of Cupid and Venus's help. Come to me, I need you as you do me, and I call you (say the name of your loved one, or the description of the person you want to come to you)*

to come to me. I request the help of Venus to take possession of (this person's pronouns) mind and (this person's pronouns) heart. Wise apple, immerse yourself and circulate through the blood of (name) so that (person's pronouns) comes and stays by my side. Come to me (person's name). Mighty spirit of the night, let (person's name) when (person's pronouns) sleeps, in dreams it is me who you find, that (person's pronouns) only has beautiful visions about me and that only my dreams of (person's pronouns) belong to me. Come to me (name or description of the person).

Afterwards, place the apple in a place where there is a lot of nature.

To Make a Person Marry You

Saint Dorothy is traditionally displayed carrying a basket of apples or sitting in an orchard. Also known as Saint Dora or Dorothea, her patronages include horticulture, brewers, brides, florists, gardeners, midwives, newlyweds, and love.

The apple is a sacred fruit for all witches. This is a magical symbol of love and is used to increase sexual charisma. This spell is so simple that you will only need a few elements.

You will need:

One red apple
Cinnamon
Patchouli oil
Clay plate
One red candle

On a Friday night, dress your candle with the patchouli oil and cinnamon. Light the candle and put the apple very close to the candlelight. Repeat the following prayer to Saint Dorothy:

By the radiance of thy holy life thou did draw. O Dorothy, I pray to you, so you with your grace and beauty make the person who

eats this apple ask me for marriage. O Saint Dorothy as fellow con-
testants you are entrusted of divine power, and divine glory. Amen.

Leave the apple with the candle until the candle has been fully consumed. Afterwards, pass this apple over your whole body while focusing on the person who you desire will ask you for marriage. Say three Hail Marys and the Saint Dorothy Prayer again.

After you perform this ritual, the person you want to marry you must eat the apple.

Garlic, Rue, Cloves, and Rosemary

Nuevo León has a mystique all its own among the states of Mexico, marked by an enduring and controversial "Jewish question" regarding its founding. Its present is as unique as its past, since although it is little known, the origin of Nuevo León, Coahuila, north of Zacatecas and Southwest Texas are interwoven with the real life drama lived by the crypto-Jews of New Spain, as it was known then.

Although it is true that there were groups of Jews who converted and genuinely adhered to Christianity, the overwhelming truth is that Crypto-Judaism (the secret practice of Judaism) was a majority trend among New Christians. The founders of Nuevo León, Mexico, were Jewish, expelled from Spain or forcibly converted to Catholicism, who suffered at the hands of the Inquisition. Two genealogical studies of the eighteenth century, the *Archivo General de la Nacion de Mexico* and the *Ramo de la Inquisition*, suggest that Father Miguel Hidalgo y Costilla, the father of Mexican Independence, had a Converso background, and that Bartolome de las Casas, a bishop who fought to free slaves in Nueva España, also had Jewish ancestors. Although as far we know, their families were sincere converts, it is ironic that expelling the Jews from Spain precipitated events that eventually led to Spain's loss of Mexico[1]. It can be deduced that during the government of Luis Carvajal

---

1 Mel Goldberg, "A Brief History of Jews in Mexico," *www.lakechapalajewishcongregation.com.*

y de La Cueva, Monterrey (the capital of Nuevo León) was a discreet Jewish colony. After the persecution, many Jews were stripped of their traditions, folklore, and identity; however, the footprint of Judaism is still present in the lives of many Mexican families.

Sephardic Jewish traditions were heavily influenced by the power of garlic, rue, cloves, and rosemary as symbols of strength, which absorb and then repel the evil. While today many people have negative connotations about garlic "stench," Jewish and Mexican people love garlic. It is one of the principal allies for Brujeria de Rancho, known for driving away bad spirits and ill intent. Garlic gives strength and is a powerful antibiotic in addition to being a powerful culinary flavor enhancer.

Rue, commonly known as *ruda* in Mexico, is seen as hugely protective, so it was planted in and around the home. Caution should be used with rue as it is toxic if ingested in more than a very small amount. Just as garlic and rosemary add flavor to a dish in addition to their magical and protective usage, so do *clavos de olor* (cloves), which can be used in multiple hechizos and rituals due their effectiveness. Rosemary is a multipurpose plant associated with remembrance, dominance, purification, and health. Below you will find some of my favorite spells utilizing these important Jewish and Mexican ingredients.

To Dominate a Specific Adversary with Garlic

You will need:

An image of Saint George
One head of garlic, unpeeled
A brown paper bag
A red pen
Your scissors
Black cloth
A piece of heavy furniture (such as a dresser, sofa, or table)

Write the name and date of birth of your enemy or adversary on the brown paper bag using your red pen. Wrap the garlic along with the image of Saint George in the black cloth and place in the brown paper bag. Take the bag with its contents and put it on the floor by your heavy furniture. Lift up the furniture and slide the garlic underneath one of its legs, then let the furniture fall on the garlic and crush it. Say the following:

> *Just as heavy as this furniture, as heavy my power and my will is over you, I crush your will, your words, your thoughts, (name of the person you wish to dominate).*

Leave the garlic underneath the heavy furniture for three days. On the fourth day, remove it from that place and throw it away in the trash.

Protection for Military Members

This spell is especially for my military family, to protect and send light to our beloved ones who serve. Since my son joined the U.S. Navy, I do this spell work every time he is deployed. It helps both of us, me to have peace of mind and heart and him to overcome any danger.

You will need:

A red candle
One prayer card of Saint Michael Archangel
Olive oil
Rosemary
Oregano
Garlic skin
A plate

On a Tuesday, preferably at night, mix the rosemary, garlic skins, and the oregano on a small plate. Anoint the candle from the tip to the base with the olive oil and sprinkle the herbs over it. Light the candle and repeat the following prayer:

> *Almighty God, let a ray of light illuminate the heart and mind of the great leaders of nations and let peace reign in the world. Heavenly God, protect my (child, friend, spouse, or parent)*

who is now in the line of duty, protect them with the shield of Saint Michael the Archangel, and keep them free from danger, may your love allow them to return home to the side of their family, I ask you on behalf of our Lord Jesus Christ. Amen.

Salación: Salting

The salación is a highly feared work of hechicería that uses salt as the main ingredient. It is carried out with the aim of killing, injuring, or financially ruining a person, a business, or a household. Being *salado* (salty) is an extremely unpleasant mental, financial, physical, moral, and spiritual state.

The salación can also make a person become financially bankrupt and unemployable, so that they cannot prosper in any aspect related to money. It can do the same for love matters. Even a house can be *salada*. If the salación is not removed, the situation can last for months, years, and even decades, with much damage to both the victim, their entire family, and other families that will come to inhabit the property in the future. salación brings calamity and misfortune to your target.

The best way to accomplish this is to drop a combination of salt mixed with other ingredients at the target's household door or business, but if you are able to do it inside their house, then that is way better. You do not need a lot of the salt mixture; with a tiny amount, you can cause great harm.

Salt of Seven Canteens
This is by far the most feared salación of all. Our grandmas used to say that we should never consume salt from a bar and instead always carry our own with us. Next time you're at a bar, try to take some of their salt and place it in a red sack. You never know when you might need it.

It is well known that salt cleans places. Salt from a bar does that too, but it also absorbs energy from its surrounding: stories and feelings of pain and sorrow. When you consume salt in that kind of business, you absorb that energy too, and you may be affected by it. Protect yourself!

> *Stolen salt from seven bars*
> *Vinegar*
> *Urine*
> *A glass container*

In preparation, go to seven different bars (preferably dive bars) and steal some salt each.

Stick it in a red sack. Once you have completed this task, place some of your urine (a few drops are enough) in a jar for seven days. On the seventh day, pour an equal proportion of salt, and let this sit for another seven days. On the fourteenth day, add seven drops of vinegar to this mixture. Let the mixture sit on the fifteenth day. On the sixteenth day, this liquid should be emptied in a cross shape outside of the target's place. (It doesn't have to be a huge cross, a tiny one is enough.) This will be enough for that home or person to remain salada for the next seven years.

Be careful, a lot of homes and businesses now have camera systems installed outside. If that's the case, you can throw the salt discreetly and form a cross with your left shoe. You can find salt from seven canteens in certain esoteric shops or botanicas, but the tradition is to steal it. If you cannot, buy it at the shop and consecrate it with your urine and vinegar.

Sal de la Viuda: Widow's Salt

To cause ruin, accidents, and injury to someone or some place, you will need:

> *Salt previously obtained from a widow (the more bitter the widow, the better)*
> *Broken glass shards from a car accident (you need to be extremely*
> *   careful collecting this because this itself contains evil*
> *   air; gloves and orifice coverings are mandatory)*
> *Cumin*

On a Tuesday, grind together the glass and the salt. The salt does not have to be a large quantity, and a single piece of glass is enough. Remember to handle broken glass carefully; not only does glass obtained from a car accident contain evil air, but most likely also sharp edges. Grind it to a powder and add the cumin while you repeat the name of your target or targets twenty-one times. Take the mixture and place it on the wheels of your target's car, on their door. Or if, for practical or legal reasons, you are unable to reach your target, introduce this mixture in a brown paper bag with a picture of your target and let it sit for thirteen days. Afterwards, discard the bag away from your home, preferably at a cemetery.

Salación with Tears for Revenge

Not all tears are the same. Tears express many emotions: love, sorrow, sadness, grief. Tears are the silent language of sadness, and a powerful weapon. In Mexican folklore, the eyes are the windows of the soul and tears bring bad luck and salación, especially those tears of sadness, hatred, and resentment. That's one of the reasons why Mexican people avoid crying at a wedding at all costs, since it is believed that those tears would bring bad luck to the new couple. To use tears to get revenge for an injustice, you will need.

> Iodized kitchen salt
> A few tears collected from the person who is suffer-
>   ing and wants revenge (they can be your own)
> Chile cascabel seeds

Crush the salt, the tears, and the chile seeds together. Repeat the following conjure:

> Spirit of justice springs from the eyes of (name of the person)
> when invoked, and its only weapon is the claim of justice coming
> out of (person's pronouns) eyes. I invoke you, so my will (or the
> will of the person you are doing this working for) be done. Make
> (person on whom you want revenge)'s life misery, ruin, and ill-
> ness. Make (person's name) dreams turn to dust. Make my whims

(person's name)'s whims and my suffering (person's pronouns) suffering, and my tears (person's pronouns) tears, so be it for this is my will. Amen.

Place this salt where you know the person is going to step into it.

CHAPTER THREE

THE SYMBOLS AND TOOLS OF TRADITION

"We hardly ever realize that we can cut anything out of our lives, anytime, in the blink of an eye."

Carlos Castaneda, *The Wheel of Time: The Shamans of Mexico, Their Thoughts About Life, Death and the Universe*

Symbols are important because they facilitate communication and identification of ideas and other concepts. Though symbols can have literal as well as figurative meanings, all communication is achieved through their use. Some symbols are used to represent elements, others to represent ideas. A foreign language has no meaning to you because you have not been given the tools to unlock its meaning. If you understand what I'm writing right now, it is because you learned symbols in order to communicate: the written language.

Since the beginning of the time, societies used some symbols to articulate the deeper concepts that they could not put into the symbols known as "words." To understand Mexican magic, you need to be able to understand the symbols we use and the reasons behind why we use certain tools. These symbols can be exchanged or replaced with others, *as long as you understand the meanings and the mechanics behind them.*

Before the arrival of the conquistadors and Christianity, sorcerers already existed in the pre-Columbian world. Though they were not like the witches of the European stories, some of these sorcerers were truly terrifying. In addition to their pre-Hispanic characteristics, over time these sorcerers were attributed Spanish traits in both origin and actions. Many of them became syncretized with Spanish beliefs and their concepts of witchcraft, attributing their abilities to demonic pacts. At the time, local towns were incredibly afraid to even speak their names out loud. These are the stories of some of the most famous Brujas de Rancho in Mexico.

The Huasteca Witch

In a ranch in the state of Veracruz, close to Copaltitla town, from 1900 to 1910 shortly before the Mexican Revolution, there was a lady named Marcelina. She was well known because she was a shapeshifter.

Marcelina's story has a depressing aspect. It was rumored that she controlled her husband with concoctions and powders. These kept him in a trance that made Marcelina beautiful in his eyes, when she was actually a thin, haggard woman with pale skin, long dirty nails, little hair, and an unbearable smell.

Marcelina lived in a remote hut surrounded by old trees with large and shadowy branches. It is said that between midnight and three AM she carried out a ritual of transformation that consisted of sprinkling aguardiente (Firewater of Agave) to prepare a fireplace in which she added agave roots, copal, and dried zoapatle leaves (also known as cihuapatli or *Montanoa tomentosa*), an herb that has a long history of use in Mexican herbal medicine to boost libido and sexual pleasure. Once the fire was ready, she jumped on it three times, from north to south and from east to west, to later sit in the direction of her victim's home. She would blow smoked copal from her mouth all over the place, making conjures and prayers in such a strange way that she even changed her voice. She would smear wet ash on her knees until she disarticulated her limbs. During that time in the village, several dead newborns were found without apparent cause or culprit.

But one night her husband returned to find his wife in full transformation. There, for the first time, he could see what she really looked like. Angry and hurt, he decided to quietly wait for her to leave and took her legs, which she had previously removed through that ritual, and went to the Sierra and buried them. After that, it is said he returned to their house and set the whole place on fire. Once Marcelina returned, she realized that her house was on fire and her legs were missing. When the first light of dawn lit that morning, she become human again, but without her legs she had to crawl on the floor. Her husband left her to die alone and mutilated.

Given how Marcelina removed her legs and the other details of the rituals she performed, we can infer that Marcelina was a Mometzcopinqui. To go deeper into Marcelina's story, I recommend listening to "La Bruja de la Huasteca," a song by the Trio Cantores del Alba.

The Sorceress of La Petaca

In northeast Mexico, about a hundred miles away from the U.S. border, lies a ranchito called Linares in the State of Nuevo León. Sorceresses are an important part of Neo-Leonese folklore. In any municipality that you visit, you will be able to hear stories involving them—many of which were used to scare us as children if we misbehaved— and these have been shared from generation to generation, even to this day.

One of the most famous stories is about a native man from the area. He was probably a member of the Cacalote tribes. This man met a witch from Querétaro state who had a granddaughter. People said that the granddaughter was the product of a demon that had impregnated the witch's daughter. While these people wanted to kill her, the Jesuits helped her and commissioned the Cacalote man to hide the witch's granddaughter and protect her.

The Cacalote man accepted, and the witch packed a suitcase for her granddaughter in which she included some strange but powerful objects and amulets to take care of the child. However, even though the man passed the girl off as his daughter, and raised her as its own, rumors began to flood the town, and so the man buried the suitcase.

Before long, people started talking about a buried devilish "petaca." That is what suitcases were colloquially called. Because of that, the town was later known as the town of La Petaca. It was said that the witch's granddaughter grew up to become a powerful and extremely beautiful sorceress. She fell in love with a boy named Macario who betrayed her, as he already had a wedding planned with another girl named Mariana. People speculated that this sorceress would turn into a crow during the nights and would hide in a *pirul* tree (pepper tree) outside Mariana's house.

Mariana was deeply in love with Macario. She did not believe in sorcery and magic, and so completely ignored the comments that people made. One day the sorceress warned Macario not to get married or bad things would happen to him, but he ignored all the threats and even dared to laugh in her face.

Finally, the day of the wedding came. Macario was waiting for Mariana in the church, but she never came. She had become extremely ill from a very rare disease and ended up dying in her white wedding gown. People whispered that at Mariana's funeral a crow was singing a song that sounded like a horrific laugh. After the funeral, the crow opened its wings and took off toward La Petaca.

Other versions of this story suggest that following the arrival of the Spaniards, the witches' spirits were locked in a petaca and buried during an exorcism, giving the town of two thousand people its name. Crosses were put up at La Petaca's four corners to ward off evil. They remain still today, as does the area's reputation as a caldron where witches cook up powerful magic.

People in all northern ranchos grew up hearing these tales about sorceress women that would transform themselves into a crow to approach and prey on their victims. For another version of this story, I recommend listening to "La Cuerva de La Petaca" by Carlos y José.

The Bruja's Scissors

One of the Brujeria de Rancho's most important teachings is that both nature and magic could not generate something new if they were forced to preserve the old. It would be like forcing a seed to never change its shape. Just as the metal had to be melted and the tree had to be cut down to create the sickle, death and transformation sustains our tools and our magic.

The reason that scissors are extremely important and emblematic in protection in Mexican folklore traces back to the Indigenous beliefs that became combined with European ones during colonial times. During pre-Hispanic times, when sorceresses like the Mometzcopinqui were captured, the most effective way to disarm them was to cut off their hair from the crown, since in this way they would lose their *tonalli* (vital force) and their powers to harm someone. This belief was documented by Jacinto de la Serna in the *Manual de Ministros de indios, para el conocimiento de sus idolatrías y extirpación de ellas* first published in 1656. De la Serna references that the pre-Hispanic population believed that a practical method used to prevent a witch from entering a location was to place an obsidian blade inside a jícara filled with water. It was said that when the witch saw herself reflected in the water, she would flee in terror. In more modern versions, the obsidian blade was substituted with scissors and the jícara filled with water was exchanged with a mirror in order to protect the population from witches.

On the other hand, the European belief suggests that many people thought scissors look not only like a cross, but also like two swords. Swords are often representative of protective figures and the fight against evil. Images of swords pointing upward historically indicate battle or the readiness for battle. Another interpretation of scissors among Brujeria de Rancho is the use of deadly spiritual force against something or someone. My grandma Diana taught me from a very young age to use the scissors like a bruja de rancho. On my seventh birthday, she gave me a beautiful 14k gold necklace strung with an already consecrated scissors pendant and a separate pair of work scissors for spell work and protection.

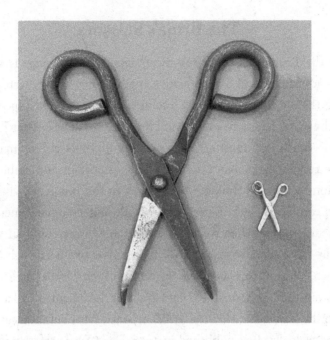

There was a funny difference between the kind of households in which some of us grew up. When we heard our elders say, "Can you hand me the good scissors, please?" that question had a totally different meaning for some of us. In that exact moment, we knew that things were going to start getting lit and that there was some business that needed to be handled.

According to Mexican folklore, scissors are protections against witches and their ill intentions. You may wonder, how do we brujas defend ourselves with a tool that, historically, had been used to harm us? To take our magic away? Well, sorcery and witchcraft in Mexico as in many other cultures, is a different experience for everyone. Although there are witches who are dedicated to benevolent matters such as healing, advisory, and other socially accepted endeavors, there were also those with sinister intents. To put it plainly, in modern terms, sometimes you may run into a situation where another witch's goals and desires oppose your work or love life—someone who wants to go after what you have—and in those cases, you need to protect yourself. This is a scenario in which you need your scissors.

Scissors are an ancient tool that is widely used in Mexican magic, a utensil that today has two purposes: to defend and to attack. Scissors are the best and most traditional tool for your work. They are useful when you want to cut something, like a relationship, an illness, a situation, but they can also be used as a barrier for protection, a boundary that says do not cross. They are also used in healing and protection work. You can hide an open pair of scissors near a sick person to cut an illness while you pray next to their bed, or wield them to protect yourself or someone else from witchcraft attacks. Scissors are traditionally used to perform powerful *limpias*. A limpia is, literally, the act of making something clean by removing dirtiness from a place or person using physical methods, spiritual methods, or a combination of the two. Scissors are also used to cut any binding work, as well to accomplish powerful ligatures (domination over your partner).

The best scissors to use are iron. Iron is often associated with the earth itself and the planet Mars, and early weaponry was made from iron ores. It is more difficult than it used to be to find iron scissors, so if you can find only steel ones, that's okay, too. Steel is an alloy made up of iron with typically a few tenths of a percent of carbon to improve its strength and fracture resistance compared to iron. Steel scissors can be used for many of the same purposes, and in fact we can view them as helping us with risky endeavors for which we need to figuratively "steel" ourselves. Make sure you use your consecrated magical scissors only for spell work or protection. Your consecrated magical scissors aren't for daily household tasks. Right now, I'm using steel scissors with red handles, and they work wonders.

The scissors are the emblem of Brujeria de Rancho or Mexican sorcery, the heraldic device and the distinctive badge. Scissors are the perfect symbol of symbiosis of cultures of our magical practices of the old and new world and all of our ancestors' beliefs about magic and the best ally to our craft. In Mexico, the meaning of scissors will always be associated with the supernatural world. The first hechizos (spells) in the colonial era were actually "spell crafted" or sewn by hand, carried in little fabric pouches and sometimes pinned or sewn on clothes. As such, scissors, needles, pins, threads, and cords are by no means random objects in Mexican magic.

Note: Never let just any person gift *tijeras* (scissors) to you. The tijeras need to be bought by you. If they are gifted, it must be done by another trusted bruja de rancho or an elder, otherwise, after they are consecrated, this pair of scissors will cause arguments, grievances, and oftentimes the breakup of a friendship or marriage. The exception to the "no gifts" rule is if you are gifted them by a witch.

To Consecrate Your Brujeria Scissors

Whether you want to wear a scissors pendant for protection or you are consecrating your spell scissors, you will need:

> *The scissors (either a scissor pendant or a pair of scissors)*
> *A Mexican clay bowl*
> *A package of fava beans*
> *Cenizo (also known as Texas sage, Leucophyllum frutescens)*
> *or estafiate (Artemisia ludoviciana).[1]*
> *Holy Water*
> *A lodestone*
> *A new rag to clean the scissors.*

The procedure is to be performed during a Dark Moon (or under a totally invisible moon) at midnight. You are going to grab your scissors with your left hand and clean them with Holy Water and a new rag. After you do this, you are going to put the scissors on your bowl along with the lodestone. Spread a package of fava beans on top of the scissors and sprinkle the cenizo leaves or estafiate around that bowl.

---

1   This herb that grow naturally in the southwestern United States or the Mexican states of Coahuila, Nuevo León, and Tamaulipas in Northern Mexico. But if not, you can use estafiate. Estafiate is the commonly used term for Artemisia ludoviciana, also called prairie sage, white sagebrush, Mexican wormwood, and Louisiana sage, or any kind of sage plant There are many different types of sage or salvia plants available. They may be either perennial or annual, blooming to nonblooming, but pretty much each of these different types of sage is fairly hardy, which is what we need.

Repeat the following prayer:

Powerful scissors, virtuous talisman, and heraldic device of rancho sorcerers, through you I ask the Lord to save me from being defeated physically or spiritually and I humbly ask that if some practitioner of witchcraft, sorcery, or any enemy of mine is plotting against me, that with the Soul of Our Lord Jesus Christ and by your power I may be armed. Make my enemies and opponents retreat while you are hanging on my house or on my neck. Make those witches, sorcerers, demons, and their animals surrender, just like the Devil surrendered to Saint Michael. Make all my invisible enemies go away and cut all their ill intentions and jealousy with your sharp edge so they do not harm me or my family or my property, cut all negativity, all vice, anger, pain, and lack of faith, bindings, laces, hexes, chains, and everything that does not allow me to prosper physically, mentally, financially, and spiritually. Amen.

After you say your prayer, you are going to take the scissors out of the bowl and leave them outside the entire night in a place where they can be exposed to the sky. Then you will to be able to wear your necklace or use your scissors for your spell work or protection for yourself. I highly encourage that you keep a red ribbon tied to the left side so you can hang them and they do not get lost. They need to be with you, at your altar if you are working or hanging on your door or window. When my grandma needed to cut an illness, she used to put her scissors next to our bed while she prayed.

Placed open to the left of your spell work, your scissors cut negative energies, bad habits, and banish people and situations away. Placed open to the right side of your spell work, they unlock situations that do not advance, and will open paths and protect. If you are using your scissors to protect your house from witchcraft, it is recommended to place them open on your window hanging on a red ribbon. If you feel that this is particularly bad moment in your life and that you could be a victim of a witchcraft attack, or you're experiencing lots of problems and difficult situations, leave the scissors wide open and place them under your bed. Once you feel that the situation has begun to change, close them, then remove them.

Hechizo Abre Caminos: Road Opener Spell

When brujos and brujas in Mexico talk about road opening works, we are talking about are endless possibilities. The roads we are speaking about are the pathways to all the good things in life: love, joy, health, prosperity, business, money, abundance, and good luck. An abre caminos (road opener) can be a spell, a ritual, or even a *baño* (spiritual bath) with spiritually prepared water. My grandma Diana used to say that an abre caminos is a form of magic all its own. Its goal is to open, to clear or create roads, the pathways to a good life full of blessings. As brujos de rancho, we are way makers. This abre caminos is designed to help open those roads for you to cut all the obstacles. Among the countless rituals that Mexicans have developed over many years, few have a significant importance as the abre caminos found below.

You will need:

One white candle or road opener prayer candle
One clear glass filled with water
Your consecrated scissors
Abre caminos oil or blessed olive oil
Estraza paper (craft paper)
Clay (barro) plate

On a Tuesday, write on your estraza (craft) paper all the areas in your life that you need help with, where you need to clear your path. You can write things like health, love, or career, to name some common examples. When you are finished, place the barro plate on top of your list. Rub your candle with the abre caminos oil or the blessed oil, or make three little holes inside your abre caminos candle and add the abre caminos oil inside of them. Light your candle and place it on top of your clay plate. Place your consecrated scissors opened to the left of your candle and place the glass of water to the right. Once your candle has burned down, remove the plate with the candle wax and grab the paper. Repeat the following prayer:

> *In the name of the Father, the Son, and the Holy Spirit, just as I cut this paper, I cut any ties, witchcraft, obstacles, and negative situations that are not aligned with success, blessings, triumph, victory, joy, happiness.*

Then cut the paper with your scissors. Once the paper is cut, repeat the following second part of the prayer:

> *In the name of the Father, the Son, and the Holy Spirit, may the doors open, may my paths be cleared, may the Divine illuminate and bless all my roads, today and forever. Amen.*

Mecate, Cords, and Knots

During pre-Hispanic times in Mexico, divination through cords and mecates (a type of reins) was a common practice. Such sorcerers were called the Mecatlapuhqui. The principal goal of this divination was to tell if a person was going to live or to die, and if they were sick, if they were going to be able to heal. When European witches and sorcerers arrived during the Mexican colonization, they brought with them their own practices involving using cords and knots for magical and healing purposes. The practice as we know it today was not only influenced by our Indigenous ancestry, but also by our Iberian ancestry.

Formerly, mecates used for divination and magic were made of ixtle. Ixtle is a stiff plant fiber obtained from a number of Mexican plants, chiefly species of agave. A strong fiber, excellent for cordage and basketwork, it evolved into the natural jute cord, which is what we use today.

Knots and cords have a special meaning in Mexican *magia* (magic)— "the cord of life" that represents human destiny. Knots are ambivalent; just as they can be tied and untied, they can be used to cause either good or evil, and serve as protection or as an attack, to symbolically tie someone in order to stop or immobilize an enemy. We can tie any type of energy into a knotted cord and hold that energy until we need it at a later date. There are so many ways to use knot magic to achieve your goals, and you can incorporate many elements such as color to reinforce intent.

There is also a wealth of folklore attached to spinning and weaving practices. The Tzitzimimeh are celestial beings who weave the destinies of people. Tlazolteotl-Ixcuina is a Mesoamerican goddess; the "Ixcuina" in her name is from the Huastec for "Goddess of Cotton." Her headdress usually includes two spindles of unspun cotton, which connect Her to weaving and to the rich cotton-growing region of the Huastec. The goddess Mayahuel, who is also primarily associated with the day sign *malinalli*, has a name often translated as "twisted grass," "grass rope," or "broom." She wears blue clothing (the color of fertility), and a headdress of spindles and unspun maguey (ixtle) fiber. The spindles on her headdress symbolize the transformation or revitalization of disorder into order and power.

Divination with Natural Jute Cord

This is a spell to prepare a mecate for divination. You will need:

> Natural jute cord (the thinner the better)
> A ruler
> Tobacco or copal to blow the offering
> Scissors
> A shawl to cover your head
> Mezcal or tequila, enough for two shots
>> (if you are underage or prefer not to use alcohol, use aguamiel)

To begin, cover your head with a shawl. Get your shot of mezcal or tequila (or aguamiel) ready to drink. Before you drink it, talk to it. Ask the spirit to guide you through your divination. Drink the first shot.

Repeat the following:

> *Mayahuel, your truth will be said. Hail Mary, I do not want it, Our Father, how good is this! Blessed [mezcal/tequila], sweet torment, what are you doing outside of me? Get inside quick.*

Then immediately take the second shot.

Now grab your scissors and your ruler. Measure the mecate and cut a twelve inch length. Give this cord to the person who seeks answers and have them tie a knot for each and every question they have. (These must be yes or no questions.) The querant must think about their questions without telling them to the diviner. Once they have thought about them, have them give the jute cord back to you. Blow some tobacco or copal as an offering to Mayahuel, and then say this prayer:

> *Mayahuel, the ones who drink from your milk get drunk. Ometochtli, those who get drunk always tell the truth. Mayahuel, I seek the Truth, whatever it may look like. Guide me, divine Goddess, and help me to always speak the Truth with a Loving tone and to move away from omissions, confusion, and anything that is not a deliberate reflection of the Truth, so I make this prayer to reveal what needs to be revealed, and help me to have knowledge of many things and not be deceived. Mayahuel, You are the Source of my voice. Amen.*

Start untying the knots one by one every time you deliver an answer to the consultant.

Mecate to Catch a Witch and Get Rid of a Maleficio

In the northeastern ranchos, our grandmothers used to tell us stories. They knew that evil exists, and that often this evil is sent as a *maleficio*. There are several types of witchcraft attacks, one of the most terrifying is the maleficio, a type of spiritual working against someone or something. Even at a distance, brujas are able to send them through rituals and sympathetic magic.

There are distinct types of shields and protections, such as Holy Water and cross-shaped scissors. However, in the ranches, there are other methods that we were taught.

Since ancient times, the best way to catch and defeat a witch is the Twelve Truths of the World cord. Most people involved in Mexican Folk Catholicism are familiar with this prayer, but not as many are aware of this ritual. The Twelve Truths have their origin in the 12th century Jewish poem *Echad Mi Yodea* ("Who Knows One?"). It is very likely that following the expulsion of the Jews from Spain, the poem was reworked with Christian content and then reached Mexico with the Anusim in the 16th century. The prayer has survived in rural areas of northeastern Mexico, along with different rituals to treat the symptoms of maleficios and get rid of their senders.

This is one of our most powerful prayers, which has been used as an exorcism. It's known colloquially as "the bruja prayer." The Twelve Truths prayer you will find below was taught orally mainly to those who worked at night and walked the roads full of dangers and las brujas de rancho.

For this work, you only need five things:

The "Twelve Truths of the World" prayer
A natural jute cord
Your spell scissors
A black candle
Matches

When detecting the slightest symptom of a hex or immediately after discovering that a bruja is after you, you must look for a natural jute cord. Be sure to have it on hand. Light the black candle while you recite the Twelve Truths of the World. Each time a truth is pronounced, tie a knot in the string. Keep tying a knot for each truth until there are twelve knots in the cord. You must remain calm; if there is any mistake in the prayer or if you become distracted, this ritual will not have any effect.

Having prayed the Twelve Truths of the World, you must say them again from memory, but in reverse order, starting with the twelfth truth and count backwards until the first. Every time you pray a truth, you undo the last knot you made in the string. Continue like this until you finish the prayer, simultaneously leaving the string without knots. You are going to burn the knotless cord with the flame from the black candle. While the cord is burning, repeat the thirteenth truth. The thirteenth truth is what our elders taught us and what makes this a witch prayer.

> *Of the twelve truths of the world, tell me the first, the holy house of Jerusalem.*

> *Of the twelve truths of the world, tell me the second, the two tablets of Moses.*

> *Of the twelve truths of the world, tell me the third, the Holy Trinity.*

> *Of the twelve truths of the world, tell me the fourth, the four gospels.*

> *Of the twelve truths of the world, tell me the fifth, the five wounds.*

> *Of the twelve truths of the world, tell me the sixth, the six candelabras.*

> *Of the twelve truths of the world, tell me the seventh, the seven words that Jesus Christ said in the Holy Wood of the Cross.*

> *Of the twelve truths of the world, tell me the eighth, the eight anguishes.*

> *Of the twelve truths of the world, tell me the ninth, the nine months of Mary.*

> *Of the twelve truths of the world, tell me the tenth, the Ten Commandments.*

> *Of the twelve truths of the world, tell me the eleventh, the eleven thousand virgins.*

Of the twelve truths of the world, tell me the twelfth, the Twelve Apostles who went with Jesus Christ from his preaching to his death on the Cross at Calvary.

Of the twelve truths of the world, tell me the thirteenth, the thirteen is the thirteen powers of Saint Michael sending this evil witch and her maleficio to burn in hell, so it shall be, in the name of the Father, the Son, and the Holy Ghost.

Amen.

If you are doing this spell for yourself, you say only the thirteen truths without saying the first part. So instead of saying "Of the twelve truths of the world, tell me," etcetera, you would only say, "The Twelve Apostles who went with Jesus Christ from his preaching to his death on the Cross at Calvary." If you are doing this for someone else, you must recite the first part of the prayer while the other person is responding. This person is in charge of tying and untying the knots. Once the prayer is done in reverse, the person should burn the cord with the candle and take the ashes to a crossroad.

To Keep a Straying Significant Other from Wandering

Infidelity and divorce were some of the things brujos de rancho combated using this ancient resource. This method works wonders with a partner who wants to "explore" outside of their relationship.

This ritual used to be more complicated, since today you can easily find out your significant other's height. Before it was this easy, brujos used to buy a couple of yards of mecate or red ribbon. When the significant other passed out on the bed, they measured them with the ribbon so it was exactly the same length as their significant other's body. Today, you can simply ask. Once you have the ribbon cut to the appropriate length, tie it around the middle of a white candle where you are going to write the name of your SO with a wooden toothpick. Turn the candle into an upside down candle by cutting off a portion of a candle where the exposed wick is, called the head, and then cut away the wax on the opposite end, called the foot, to expose the wick on that end. This is how you are going to burn the candle. Burn it every night until it is consumed to the middle where the ribbon is tied (it doesn't have to be a huge candle). Once the candle is consumed to the middle, you are going to untie the ribbon and place a Saint Anthony medal on it. Roll it up and carry it with you always. The rest of the candle must be hidden in your underwear drawer. You can wear the ribbon as a bracelet on your dominant hand, but be aware you are carrying someone's leash with you, so you can't misplace it or lose it.

Amarres

Amarre literally means "mooring" in Spanish, a ligature or knot that holds two or more elements together. The practice is an imitative or sympathetic ritual of marriage ceremonies in Mexico. The idea behind sympathetic rituals is, at its core, that a person can be affected magically by actions performed toward something that represents those spiritual ceremonies. Sympathetic magic is a magical modality that involves symbolically imitating the desired outcome. In this case, the pre-Hispanic ceremony known as the *Amarre de Tilma y Huipil* (mooring of the tilma and huipil), which was performed to unite young Mexica couples in marriage. The mooring of tilma and huipil was full of symbolism, where a spiritual promise arose between two souls who wanted to form a unity for eternity: in the here-now and in the hereafter. During the union ritual, the woman wore a huipil and the man a tilma, clothing that was tied by the Mexica priest.

With the arrival of the Spaniards, a syncretism was made between the Catholic and this ancestral practice. A large percentage of Mexicans are Catholic or Folk Catholic, but there is still a lot of social pressure to get married by the Catholic Church and have a traditional wedding. At a Mexican wedding, the *lazo* (lasso), which is associated with a wedding prayer during the ceremony, visually represents the unbreakable bond between the bride and groom. That force unites them and sets them apart from the rest of the world, protecting them and invigorating their alliance. Today, the tradition of the lazo continues to make its way around the world. In 2013, it was officially recognized in the United States as part of the Catholic marriage ceremony. Its depth will never be extinguished, since it lies in its own name: in Spanish, as in Sanskrit, the word *yug* means bond and ties at the same time.

An amarre in magic is a spell to dominate, control, and seduce. It is used to make someone believe to fall in love, to tie someone to another person whether they want it or not. This is by far one of the most iconic and feared practices in Mexican Brujeria: an amarre you tie on a specific person without consent, depriving them of their free will.

Here's my take: yes, amarres are a form of magical manipulation and coercion in the 2022 lens, but so are Instagram filters, putting on make-up, dying hair, lip fillers, choosing fancy restaurants for dates that don't match with financial solvency and paying with credit cards that we are not even able to pay back, the simple act of flirting or trying to make someone laugh—they are all forms of manipulation. In every case, we are trying to make someone feel good about us, to make them feel an attraction, to like us, to think about us, and ultimately feel love for us. Ethical or unethical? That's not my job to decide. At the end of the day, we create our own excuses and justifications.

As a bruja de rancho, I get it: desperate times call for desperate measures. There is only one thing I say to every woman or man coming to me to look for an amarre, and it is this: Are you willing to risk meeting and being with the love of your life, the one is destined for you and only you, to be tied to this person? Because an amarres works both ways. Sleep on it, and come back the next day. I can tell you that I could be very persuasive, but in this case I don't push any client's decision, and 95% come back the next day. The motives are always different, and some of them are really sad. In 2022, the stigma surrounding divorce is still tied to our culture.

I've received a lot of questions because people don't seem to understand the roots, folklore, and mechanics around amarres in Mexico. Traditionally speaking, you need cords to do an amarre. There are a lot of brujas today who only use amarre in liquid forms, such as prepared liquid potions available at the botanica, small bottles with *Amarre Haitano* written on their parchment. These forms of amarres are not traditional by any means.

Amarre de las Tres Vueltas: Amarre of the Three Spins
This is by far my favorite amarre, because it is simple, inexpensive, and very effective.

You will need:

Two plain white seven-day glass candles
A picture of the couple you need to tie together (it can be two
      separate pictures, one of you or the person you are doing
      the amarre for and one of the target of the amarre)
Glue
Red cord
A permanent marker
Orange blossoms, gardenia flowers, or jasmine flowers
Rice (a very small handful will do)
Holy Water
Cinnamon stick
Mexican clay plate

This amarre must be done on a Friday. Gather all the ingredients together. Glue the pictures to the candles: one person on each candle. Once the glue is dried, write the name and date of birth of each person on the back of the candle with a permanent marker. When the candles are ready, put the flowers on a Mexican clay plate.

Place the two candles on top of the plate with the flowers. Grab your red ribbon and wrap the two candles together three times, making three turns with the ribbon. Make three knots and repeat the following:

In the name of the Father, the Son, and the Holy Ghost, with
   me you were intertwined three times, and you get tangled up more

and more. The number of times you leave my side will be the same
number of times that you will come back to me. We are tangled up
forever, intertwined with the help of our creator, now you are mine,
until the day you die. Amen.

You can change the wording of the prayer if you are doing this amarre on someone else's behalf; simply say the name of the person you are doing the amarre for and their intended. Sprinkle Holy Water on the candles with your cinnamon stick. Light the candles and repeat the following as they burn: *May the Eternal Father keep us united in love forever!*

When the candles are still lit but about to burn out, throw a little bit of rice on the candles. Once the candles have burned, remove the ribbon. Throw away the waste and buy a potted plant. Hide the ribbon in the soil and care for the plant.

Amarre de Miel: Honey Amarre

This is another example of a traditional and very simple amarre. You will need:

> One yard of red ribbon
> Two figural candles or two fetiches representing the two people to tie together
> Permanent marker
> Honey
> Three drops of your own blood
> Dried hibiscus flowers, red rose petals, and orange blossoms
> One small glass container
> One Amarre de Amor candle or red taper candle
> One toothpick
> Clay plate

Divide the red ribbon in two and on each half write the name of the targets. You must include a last name. For a man and a woman, use the last name of the man for both people, and for a same sex couple exchange their last names. Tie the figural representations of the couple with the ribbon.

In the small glass container, add three tablespoons of honey, a pinch of all three flowers, and three drops of your blood. Mix it well with the toothpick.

Once you have your mixture, use your ring finger to spread the mixture on the figural representations. Make sure to spread the mixture on the ribbon as well. Put the figural representations on top of your clay plate. Light the red candle close to the figural representations, but do not light the figural representations themselves. The candle should be a safe distance away; we are not trying to burn the figural representations.

Repeat the following prayer:

> Spirit, body, and soul of (name of the target), come to me because I call you, I dominate you. I am (your name) and you are mine now. By the dominant spirit, I dominate you in body, soul, mind, and heart. I dominate your judgment and thought, so that you are only mine and no one else's. You will never look at anyone but me, my eyes seduce you, and the words on my lips are orders for you. You are tied to me now, you are only for me from head to toe, vein for vein, nerve for nerve, meek and humbled. Spirit of dominion grant me that (name of person) has no peace but by my side, that (person's pronouns) does not fall asleep if it is not with me, that (person's pronouns) thirst and hunger is satiated only by my side.
>
> Make (person's pronouns) come desperate, imploring at my feet, begging for love, wishing to see me, full of passion for me, humble, repentant.
>
> I am (your name). Aid me, spirit of despair, and intercede by bending the five senses of (name of person) so (person's pronouns) submits to my will, so that I am the owner of (person's pronouns) faith, love, and will. To you, dominant spirit that with your divine power given by God, make (name of person) be dominated by my body and my soul; that (person's pronouns) life is not (person's pronouns) life if not by my side, that (person's pronouns) does not

approach anyone but me, that I am the only owner of (person's pronouns) love and affection. With two I see you, with three I tie you. I take my own blood to split your heart and put myself inside of it. Amen.

This prayer should be prayed for nine consecutive days beginning on a Friday.

Bracelet of the Seven Psalms: Get Rid of Enemies, Envy, and Persecutions
The Seven Penitential Psalms or the Psalms of Confession are the names for Psalms 6, 31, 37, 50, 101, 129, and 142 (6, 32, 38, 51, 102, 130, and 143 in the Hebrew numbering). These psalms were written by King David as he expressed the contrition and sorrow he felt for sins committed and his desire to amend his life, hence the title "Penitential."

You will need:

Three 17-inch purple ribbons
A lock of hair (your own if you are conducting this spell for yourself;
    otherwise use the hair of the person you are trying to protect)
A small crucifix pendant
Holy Water
Matches

Put the three ribbons together and make a knot at one end so you start braiding them along with the lock of hair. Once you finish the braid, tie the crucifix pendant into the finishing knot. Sprinkle Holy Water on the bracelet and pray the following Seven Psalms Prayer.

I surrender myself to the Great Power of God, into the arms of Mary, the Most Holy, at the Seven Psalms and the Holy Trinity, Father, Son, and Holy Spirit. I offer myself to the three laces with which they tied Our Lord Jesus Christ on the Cross before he got nailed and crucified. With these same laces all my enemies will be tied up, from the hands to the feet. Jesus, deliver me from diabolical

*arts, deliver me from a vigorous bullet and of every cutting weapon
and free me as well from the evil temptations. I entrust myself to
the Seven Psalms, and the Angels of Heaven, so that I will not be
imprisoned nor my veins corrupted, so that my enemies do not chase
me with slander or entanglement and make my adversaries come
humble to my feet, how our Lord came at the foot of the Cross to
die. Amen.*

After you say this prayer, tie the bracelet on your left wrist and cut the excess.

To Bind an Enemy
You will need:

A photograph of your enemy
A black candle
Black ink
Black pepper
Chile cascabel seeds
Olive oil
Black ribbon or natural jute cord
Mexican clay plate

Focus on your enemy and write the name of the person and their date
of birth on the back of the picture. Take a toothpick and write their name
on the candle as well. Anoint the candle with oil and roll the candle on the
pepper and chile seeds. Tie the black ribbon around the photo, focusing on
the eyes and the mouth. Wrap it around the photo three times. As you do
this, say the following prayer:

> *I bind you, and I bind all of your thoughts, so you are not
> able to think about me, I bind you, and I bind all your words, so
> you are not able to gossip about me, I bind you and I bind your
> actions, so you can't do anything against me, I bind you from
> behind, so you do not see me come, I bind you from before, so you*

never hold me back, and not even Mary, the Undoer of Knots,
would be able to untie this knot. Amen.

Tie a really tight knot. Put the picture on a Mexican clay plate and place the candle on top of the picture. Light the candle and let it consume.

To Cross Paths with the Ideal Partner and Pull Them to Us

This is one of my personal favorite hechizos because it brought my husband to me. It is from my grandma's personal arsenal of spells. This hechizo is famous for bringing so many couples together in happy marriages. One important note: before you embark on this hechizo, it is important to know what is it is that you want in a significant other. If we don't know what we want, how can we attract them and manifest them into our lives? Get ready with your paper and pen and write a list with everything you desire in your perfect match: eye color, height, income, interests, and "other attributes" (if you know, you know!). Even if you think something is trivial, superficial, or that you are "just being picky," include it! This is Brujeria de Rancho, so do not limit yourself! As my grandmother used to say, "If you are going ask, ask good and ask enough!"

For this hechizo, you are going to need:

Your perfect partner list
Red ribbon or mecate.
Saint Anthony holy card or image
Holy Water
One pink candle or a Saint Anthony prayer candle
Blessed olive oil or patchouli oil

First, write out your perfect partner list and check it twice (or more) to make sure it includes everything that you want. Be very specific! Once you're sure your list includes everything you desire in a partner, you are going to leave it under a lit Saint Anthony prayer candle until the candle is completely consumed. (We don't want the paper to burn, so make sure you separate it from the burning candle by placing something, like a plate, between them.)

When the candle has been consumed, fold your paper three times. With each fold, repeat:

In the name of the Father, the Son, and the Holy Ghost. Amen.

If your Saint Anthony prayer card is laminated or in plastic, clean it with Holy Water. (If the card is unlaminated, do not get it wet.) Pair your prayer card and your list together. Tie a crossroad or parcel knot by taking sixteen inches of string and laying it flat across the center and top of the holy card and list. Bring the pieces all the way to the bottom and then do a half twist so they curve around one another and off to the right. Tie your knot on the top side. Once you've brought the two ends of the string back around, poke them both under the central string so that they both run parallel with a slight gap between them. Make one string U-turn back over the central string, then do the same with the other tail so that both ends lie above the opposite tail. Pulls the tails and then tie it like a shoelace. Make sure your string doesn't have any slack and your spell is almost done! Ask Saint Anthony to find this person for you and tie you together. Every Friday—the day of Venus—rub a little bit of patchouli oil on your spell. Carry this with you always, tucked into your wallet or purse.

Once you have your significant other and have formalized your relationship, continue to keep this trabajo safe, and rub it one Friday a month with patchouli oil.

CHAPTER FOUR

AMULETS AND TALISMANS

La Magia está en los detalles.
Magic is in the little details.

—Mexican folk saying

When a person finds a coin on the ground, they generally think it will be a particularly good day in terms of luck. Maybe if this same person sees a feather instead of a coin, they will think that an angel is close by. This type of belief has its origin in our ancient history, when man began to have contact with higher entities or forces. This process of belief has a long and difficult path. Even today, understanding that there are powerful forces that can help us in both spiritual and mundane matters is something that many people believe is either out of reach or simply too incredible.

You may wonder things like, is it possible that if I carry an amulet or talisman or even a sacramental object, my luck will change? Will I be protected by these simple yet complex objects?

These questions have two very simple and honest answers: Yes and no.

Surely, if you prepare your amulet or a talisman without having the knowledge to prepare it according to your needs, your amulet or talisman will only serve you as a decorative item, an accessory whose main function is to look beautiful. To create an amulet or talisman that is truly capable of protecting you, you must first have knowledge.

In this chapter, I present a wide variety of knowledge about Brujeria de Rancho amulets, along with how to design and create them, along with the talismans that we use in Brujeria de Rancho, their meanings, their power, how you can activate them, and work with them.

In Mexican magia, *amuletos* are a must. Rather than simply giving you a bunch of recipes, I want to offer you the mechanics and the freedom to create your own Mexican magical amulets. I have said several times that Mexican magic is extremely linked to the land where we live. As a practice, it is characterized by its efficiency and practicality. The herbs, stones and components that form these amulets are sacred to and shared by a group of people who find their most important meanings, symbols, and faith in those components. These amulets have changed and evolved over time. As a collector of books on brujeria and hechicería-inspired grimoires that were confiscated from practicing witches in Yucatan, Coahuila, Durango, and other states during the Mexican Inquisition, I can tell you that the amulets that were described in those texts and what today's botanicas offer differ vastly. We must keep in mind that our magic is a living and dynamic reality that is always changing, and yet it keeps the same mechanics.

Amuletos: Amulets

Many people confuse amulets with talismans. In Mexican magical terms, it is of the utmost importance that you know the difference between these two. The word amulet comes from the Latin *amuletum*, and in Mexican magic the term is used to name an object that protects us against illnesses or misadventures, or attracts certain events or situations. Generally speaking, the majority of the amulet's components are organic and come from the vegetable or animal kingdom. They are *morralitos*, little fabric bags that are filled with stones, herbs, grains, seeds, images of saints, written prayers, hair, or even animal parts like a rattle or snake skin. These sachets can serve many different purposes. The elements of an amulet are varied, but it is important that they possess certain characteristics determined according to the wearer's needs.

Our grandmas in Mexico often say "La Magia esta en los detalles," which means "the magic is in the little details." This is exactly what they mean, like a secret code word. A small bag can have a great influence on our lives. Amulets protect us and take care of our needs. Something as small as an amulet has the power to change and modify fate at our convenience. Small doses of magic manage to move mountains.

To create your amulet, you are going to need:

Colored fabric, preferably lightweight woven cotton or rayon.
    (The color of the bag corresponds to the purpose and intention of
      the amulet. You can also sometimes buy pre-made morralitos.)
Natural jute cord or string
Scissors
Herbs, seeds, grains (we are going to use materials you
    most likely already have in your pantry)
Medals, old pendants, flexible prayer cards, or images of saints

First, you must decide on the purpose of your amulet. What is it that you need? Protection? Healing? To draw love or money? Once you have decided, check the table of color correspondences in the back of this book to decide what color fabric you are going to use and the day on which you should create your amulet. You can either sew a 2x2 inch morralito yourself or you can buy one pre-made. Next, decide which herbs, seeds, and stones you are going to put inside. You do not have to put a lot of things inside your morralito; it is better to add a few things that are meaningful to you and that are carefully chosen according to the specific purpose of this amulet.

For love: cinnamon, patchouli, rose petals, High John the Conqueror root, musk, tobacco, coriander, carnation petals, lavender, nutmeg. My grandma particularly always used rice and orange blossom. In case your love life needs more passion or excitement, use hibiscus flower, Jamaica cloves, saffron, parsley, damiana, or piloncillo.

For protection: oregano, rosemary, red and black pepper, coins, salt, garlic, bay leaves, thyme, rosemary, bay, mint, alum stone, fennel seeds, mustard seeds.

For prosperity: grains and seeds, corn, bay leaf, rosemary, sandalwood, rue. Lentils and rice are a must for money matters.

Once you have chosen your herbs, seeds, and stones, look for a small object that represents your needs. If you want to get married, add a wedding ring. If you want to move house, or you are looking to improve your living conditions, you can add in a tiny piece of brick or wood. If you want to attract money add a coin The possibilities are endless, so don't limit yourself. Be creative!

Next, choose the saint, folk saint, or animal spirit to whom this amulet will be consecrated. Animal spirits are a good choice if you do not currently feel comfortable working with a saint.

A note on the prayers contained in this section: Feel free to modify (or create from scratch) your own prayers to better personalize your amulet to your specific needs or purposes. If a prayer is not resonating with you, be creative, and use a prayer with which you are comfortable and secure. Remember that this is *your* amulet that you will be carrying on your person and it must suit your needs.

Now you are ready to fill your bag. Make sure the number of elements that will fit inside is equal to an odd number—three, five, or seven. This is a very important principle in Mexican magic, as odd numbers have a great importance in Mexican folklore. Odd numbers are associated with magic and supernatural beliefs. To this day in Mexico, people still say that the first granddaughter of a bruja is consecrated to the devil. According to some beliefs, Jesus Christ died at 3 PM, and as such a lot of brujeria in Mexico is done at 3 AM, which we call the devil's hour. Oral tradition has it that the seventh child of a family is destined to become curandero/curandera, a folk healer. The number seven holds great power, especially in Brujeria de Rancho. God created the world in seven days, there are seven classical planets in astrology, seven archangels, and seven capital sins. The number seven also frequently appears in the Bible: the seven-branched candlestick, the seven spirits resting on Joseph's rod, the seven heavens where the angelic orders live, and Solomon who built the Temple in seven years. As such, numbers like three and seven have a long history in the oral traditions of Mexican magic.

Once you have finished filling your amulet with ingredients, close the bag with a string and tie three knots. Pray the Sign of the Cross prayer three times, one time for each knot on the cord. Cut the excess string. Carefully scorch the ends of your cord so that the strings will not open. Remember your fire safety! Be careful not to burn the amulet or yourself. As a final step, spray your own perfume or cologne on the amulet to disguise the smell.

For this amulet to work, you will always carry it with you. It is useless if it is left forgotten at home. Wear it hidden in your clothes so that no one can see it. In addition to the ingredients inside, the location worn on your body is also important. The *Yōllōtl* (heart) is a hugely important symbol in the pre-Hispanic rituals that endure, strong and vibrant, and remain relevant to this day. The heart is associated with love amulets. Traditionally, this symbolism is reinforced by carrying the amulets on the left side of the body. Do so for love amulets and those for protection, to keep us safe and free of harm. Amulets for prosperity, money, and luck should conversely be carried on the right side of your body.

Abundance Amulet

You will need:

A green morralito
String
Scissors
Matches
White rice
Corn
Lentils
Pinto beans

Bay leaves

An image of Saint Jude (either a medal or an unlaminated prayer card)

One coin in current circulation

On a Thursday, fill a green morralito with the rice, corn, lentils, pinto beans, bay leaves, and a coin. Fold the image or holy card three times and add it to the bag. After that, say the follower prayer (remember that you can substitute or create your own prayer!):

> *Most holy Apostle, Saint Jude Thaddeus, friend of Jesus, I place myself in your care at this difficult time. Help me know that I need not face my troubles alone. Please join me in my need, asking God to bless me with prosperity and abundance, so that I will be free from poverty, debt, and need, that you, Saint Jude, provide me with good luck and opportunities, that I will make sure to take advantage of and share those blessings with others as well, that the star of good luck shine for me and may fortune and success smile at me in all that I am set out to do. Under your patronage and grace, I place myself and all of my projects. Saint Jude, do not forsake me and always be by my side. Amen.*

Use the string to tie the bag closed and tie three knots. Pray the Sign of the Cross three times, one for each knot. Burn the loose ends of the cord with a match (be careful not to burn the bag or yourself). Afterwards, spray the bag with a little perfume or cologne. Carry it with you hidden and pinned on your right side.

Amulet to Attract True Love and Marriage

You will need:

Pink morralito

String

Scissors

A bowl

Prayer card, medal, or image of Saint Anthony of Padua
A new ring
A lock of your own hair
Rice
Cinnamon
Dry white flower petals (preferably from a white lily)
A chunk of piloncillo
Red cloth

On a Friday, place the ring in the bowl. Cover it with rice and cinnamon. On top of this, place the medal or image of Saint Anthony, and then cover the bowl with red cloth. Place the covered bowl on your altar or by your bedside for the next thirteen days. Each night for those thirteen days, say the following prayer:

> *Beloved and blessed Saint Anthony of Padua, you who are full of love, grace, generosity, and a number of beautiful qualities that God granted to you so that you could perform miracles to all those who are in great need and ask for your help. I come to you this night because you are a well-known ally of the people who request your help in love, friendship, and marriage matters, because you are a pious and generous being to all of us who are looking for love in our lives. I ask you to bring me the blessing of getting in my life my true love, a person who loves me, who will accompany me forever and who is by my side in the best and worst moments.*
>
> *That this person be my ideal person, and we complement each other, and that this person feels the love that I feel for you. I ask you to help me get the person that is going to be my partner and companion, the person that is missing in my life so we can be happy and form a family where love, understanding, joy, and unity reign. I ask you to listen to my need and help me in this task. Amen.*

On the thirteenth night, after you have finished saying your prayer, proceed to fill your pink morralito with a little bit of that rice. At this point, take the ring and wrap a lock of your hair around it before placing it in the bag. Add the medal or prayer card, flower petals, and a little chunk of the piloncillo. Tie the morralito together with the natural jute cord, making three knots at the end and praying the Sign of the Cross prayer for each knot. Sprinkle some of your perfume or cologne over the morralito. Carry this amulet on your left side.

Borreguito de la Abundancia: Abundance's Lucky Sheep

December holidays are a big deal in Mexico. People wish each other positive things such as luck, fortune, and health. On several occasions these wishes are increased or strengthened with objects that, according to popular belief, help to attract good fortune, prosperity, and abundance.

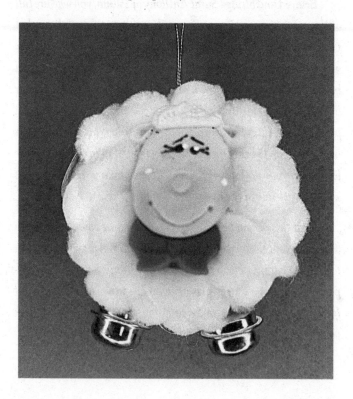

Among these objects are the so-called lucky sheep, which are characterized by their bulky wool and mischievous, cute faces, and which, on special occasions, are usually accompanied by small coins, bells, ribbons, and seeds, especially lentils. These cute little animals' origin is attributed to a legend that comes from the Swiss Alps, where this animal is considered a symbol of abundance and prosperity. That same legend emigrated to Coahuila during the 1800s when this city was an important center of commerce in the north of the country, and the states of Texas, New Mexico, Arizona, and California still belonged to Mexico. At that time, the *sarapes* that were marketed in the north of the country were from different regions, as well as those that were already manufactured in the city. However, the sarapes created in Saltillo were beginning to stand out for their characteristics. They were manufactured with a higher quality and fine wool thread, and wool became a symbol of prosperity, abundance, and money in that region.

Most of us Mexican brujas believe in "reaping what you sow." As such, it's easy to realize why this luck-bringing lamb must be given to friends and family. By giving this gift, in addition to generating greater luck for the recipient, the giver also brings good luck to themselves! That makes this lamb a perfect gift for Christmas. The sheep can be made from any material: glass, plastic, metal, fabric, or wood. Some people wear their lucky lambs as a bracelet during the New Year's dinner and the first month of January.

I have often been asked, "Can we buy a lucky lamb for ourselves?" Yes, we can! And it will still bring prosperity and abundance if we follow this ritual. I am also often asked what happens to the lamb from previous years? Can you save them and re-use them again in the new year? Of course you can, just clean them and perform the ritual again.

Once we receive a lamb (either from others or from ourselves), it should be placed on a plate with lentils and with a white or Divine Providence prayer candle. Now, you are ready to perform your ritual.

You will need:

A plate (I usually use Mexican clay materials to place my
    hechizos but you can use a clear plastic or white plate)
The borrego (sheep)
Three coins (they can be any type, even pennies, but it is
    important that they be real metal and not plastic)
A ribbon for the lamb's neck (traditionally a red ribbon, but you can use other
    colors to call abundance and prosperity in other areas of your household)
A white or Divina Providencia candle
Abrecamino oil
Dried lentils
Mustard seeds
Rosemary
Basil
A cleaning rag
Holy Water

Grab the rag and Holy Water and take all the dust of the lamb along with any attachments or ill intent from the person who gave it to you. Once it is clean, proceed to rub a little bit of abrecamino oil on your lamb while praying the Lord's Prayer three times. Place a handful or two of lentils on the plate; you want enough to cover the plate well. Fix your candle with the oil and the herbs. Place your lamb and your fixed candle on top of the plate. (You will need a big plate if you have a lot of lambs.) Take the three coins and place them on the plate in the form of a triangle.

Light the candle at the same time your family gathers to have dinner. Pray the Divine Providence prayer. If you are the only one following the ritual, you can repeat this prayer in silence.

> *Oh Divine Providence, grant me Your mercy and Your infinite*
> *goodness! Kneeling at your plants, I ask of You charity. I ask you for*
> *mine: house, clothing, and sustenance. Grant them health and take*
> *them on the right track and may it always be virtue, the one that*

guides them in their destiny. You are all my hope. You are my comfort, I believe in You, I hope in You, and I trust in You. Your Divine Providence may be extended at every moment, so that we never miss: house, clothing, and sustenance, nor the holy Sacraments at the last moment. Amen.

To receive the new year, once the candle is consumed, put your lamb near the door, preferably hanging on the doorknob during the week of the new year. With this, we ensure that money enters our house every month. Leave the lamb there for the whole month of January and then save it to re-use next year. You can place as many lambs on your lentil plate and your doorknob as you like; many people use them as decorations for their New Year's parties.

At the time of giving or receiving the sheep as a present, the following phrase should be said: *Borreguito de la montaña, has que con tu lana junte dinero cada mañana.* In English, this translates: *Little mountain sheep, have your wool give money every morning.* "Lana" (wool) is a commonly used slang term for money in Mexico, especially Northern Mexico.

Ocote Cross Amulet

The Montezuma pine (Pinus montezumae) is native to Mexico and Central America, where it is known as ocote. The word *ocote* comes from the Nahuatl word *ocotl*. In Mexico, this tree is found in states such as Nuevo León, Veracruz, and Jalisco, and is used to ward off any hexes.

It is easy to find ocote at Mexican carniceria (butcher shops) in the U.S. If you think that you are experiencing an enemy's witchcraft attack, it is advisable to put an ocote cross in the window of your room, as well as at your bedroom door and at the main door of your house. There are also small ocote crosses that you can wear around your neck.

To make your ocote cross amulet, you will need:

Three ocote sticks
One red string or ribbon

On a Tuesday, take the three ocote sticks and hold them with your left hand while praying the Lord's Prayer. Tie two of the sticks together in the form of the cross using the red ribbon or string. Once this is done, light one end of the remaining ocote stick and allow it to burn. Repeat the following prayer:

> Lord, bless this ocote so that nothing and no one can harm us. May this cross drive away the wicked, their maledictions, and their sinister intentions. May everything that is not aligned with you, my Lord, be unable to approach this place because You live in it. We trust your protection through this blessed ocote cross, which from now on will be our shield of holy protection and will be in (our home/with me) every day, making (us/me) feel your presence that accompanies (us/me) daily. You are (our/my) refuge and strength. Amen.

You can burn the whole stick or only a part of it. Once you finish this prayer, your cross is ready. For protection, burn additional ocote on Tuesdays.

Azabache Stone

Azabache is a protective amulet made from jet, a black organic rock that forms when pieces of woody material are buried in sediment and coalified. Jet is highly prized for its magical and protective properties. This Mexican belief originated from the heavy magical influences in the Iberian Peninsula. Various amulets have been made from this stone, including the azabache hand. The azabache hand is an important part of Mexican culture. It is believed to have various properties that protect from the Evil Eye, jealousy, envy, and ill intentions.

This is not the type of semi-precious stone that we see in fashion magazines, in current jewelry trends or on celebrities. It is a stone that, with composure, has entered our houses and become the guardian of our Mexican babies. Traditionally, bracelets made from azabache stone are gifted by a family member or friend, typically the *abuelitas* (grandmothers). This gift consists of a gold bracelet or necklace with a black or red coral and a charm in the form of a fist. It is believed that this gift will protect the child from the Evil Eye. Since I was a child, my family has always encouraged everyone in our household to wear an azabache bracelet.

Azabache stones can be worn as necklaces as well as bracelets. There is no need to consecrate the stone. Wear it for your protection. The stone is so powerful that there is no need for it. Traditionally, if the azabache hand or stone cracks or breaks, that means it has absorbed negative energies and done its job to repel them away from you.

The Lucky Elephant Spirit

The elephant is a symbol of luck, associated with good fortune. Elephant amulets are popular in Mexico, where the elephant is seen as a hardworking animal, symbolizing power and unity. Other connotations, such as abundance and prosperity, are also attributed to the elephant.

When using the elephant as an amulet, the trunk must always be up, and the elephant should be a white or metallic color such as silver or gold. The elephant amulet is used as a protective element for people, but especially for businesses and households. Placed facing the main entrance, the elephant brings luck, wealth, and protection.

On the seventh day of each month, put a piece of your country's currency in the elephant's trunk. For example, 10 pesos or a $10 bill. Fold the bill in seven lengthwise and say the following: *May this bill be multiplied by seventy times seven.*

Tuck the bill into the elephant's trunk. Remember that on the seventh of the following month, you must exchange that bill for a new one and follow the same steps. Do this every month so that money is not lacking in your home or business. For this amulet to continue working, take the old bills from the elephant's trunk when you exchange them and spend them at home or in your business.

Colmillo de Siete Elefantes: Seven Lucky Elephant's Tusk

For thousands of years, the seven elephants have been a symbol of good luck not just in Mexico but in many cultures throughout the world. In these representations, their tusks are usually considered symbols of power and strength.

This amulet, which takes the form of a metallic gold or silver elephant tusk engraved with the image of a herd of elephants going from largest to smallest, can be used as a road opener. To activate it, rub abre caminos oil on the metal tusk on the seventh day of the month. Burn a silver or gold candle (it should match the color of your metal elephant tusk amulet) next to your elephant tusk for seven hours.

Talismans

The word *talisman* is derived from the Greek root *teleo*, which means "to consecrate." It is precisely the ritual of consecration that gives talismans their magical powers. These objects are ascribed with magical powers, and wonderful virtues once they have been consecrated for a specific purpose. Talismans are closely linked with amulets, fulfilling many of the same roles, but a key difference is in their form and materiality. Talismans must be charged with the forces they are intended to represent, forces highly linked to planetary or elemental powers. It can be said that a talisman is an amulet in its highest stage of evolution.

Talismans in Mexican magic have been highly influenced by the Chaldeans, Egyptians, and so many other cultures. Talismans are important because they hide cultural symbols and practices that allow you to understand how an ancient practice has evolved over time, in the sense that they're no longer specific to one culture. Even though they are considered communal or cultural in nature, you must be aware that the magical power of a talisman can be overshadowed only by another talisman of greater strength or virtue, as well as the wearer of it.

A talisman requires much more elaborate work than an amulet, and for the same reason it can have a greater and more powerful influence to help you achieve your desires and aid you in the proper channeling and use of these forces. In the correspondences chapter, I provide some astrological correspondences to take into consideration, such as colors, days, and planetary hours that will help you to consecrate your talismans. It needs to be said that, while you can find any talisman made from any material or colors today, the materials used in the past used to be totally related to planetary influence.

You do not need to own an expensive talisman made from precious metals or stones for your talisman to work. There are certain talismans that in the past were crafted from lead or mercury; we know now that these materials are not safe to handle or wear. This is why magic evolves around reason and practicalities. Brujeria de Rancho is about the mechanics; as long as you understand the mechanics behind an object, taking into account the elements and the language of magic, it can be used as a talisman.

For any talisman to function properly, it is important to touch them with a lodestone or, if you cannot get a lodestone, a magnet, before using them. The universe and magic are governed by the law of attraction. Sorcerers and Kabbalists have throughout the ages known this, which is why they used lodestones to activate talismans. A lodestone is a very powerful, naturally magnetized piece of the mineral magnetite. It will work with you to attract or repel, depending on what you need. Lodestone in Spanish means *piedra imán*. Translated more accurately, piedra imán actually means magnet stone. As nouns, the difference between magnets and lodestones is that a magnet is a piece of material that attracts some metals by magnetism, while a lodestone is a naturally occurring magnet, a living being. What is the key word in both cases? Attraction! So let's work with what you have, but I highly encourage you to get the lodestone if you are able, since that is the traditional way. If you can't, use a magnet.

The first thing you are going to do if you are using a lodestone is check if it is alive. In this case, alive means that it is attracting. Usually, male lodestones attract more than female stones, but as long it is alive, it's good to work. After you know that is alive, the next step it is to clean your lodestone or magnet with Holy Water and a new rag. Make sure after you wipe it down that it is completely dry, as both lodestones and magnets tend to rust. Sprinkle a pinch of salt over it and choose a name for your lodestone. Keep in mind that this is a living being. After you have chosen a name, say the following prayer:

> *Heavenly Father, thank you for every good and perfect gift that comes from you. May this lodestone/magnet, (name of your stone), be filled with your Holy Spirit, that it may remain faithful to your power. Prepare it for the blessings and the battles to come and be my biggest ally in the tasks that I need it, (name of the stone), to fulfill. May your strength be its strength when times are hard. May its presence be full of your presence. In the name of the Father, the Son, and the Holy Spirit. Amen.*

The name that you choose for your piedra imán must be kept secret. My grandma left hers to me and my sister when she died, and I didn't know the names of her lodestones until she passed.

You have to clean and feed your lodestone or magnet every time you use it and on the first day of every month. Use magnetic sand, iron filings, or steel filings to feed your lodestone. The rancho tradition is to place your lodestone in a clay bowl with wheat seeds surrounding the lodestone.

Talismans in Mexican folk magic can be worn on a necklace or hung in your home or business. The following are the must-have talismans for Brujeria de Rancho:

Tetragrammaton

A tetragrammaton is a very famous talisman in Mexican magia, and especially in my personal practice because it represents my family tradition. My tetragrammaton has been in the family for three generations, starting with my grandma, then my mom, and now me. The tetragrammaton is used in magic as one of ineffable names of power. It is a five-pointed star around four Hebrew letters, YHVH (Yod, Heh, Vav, Heh), and planetary symbols. It is one of the most powerful talismans, enclosed with deep secrets of protection. You can find them made from different materials, ranging from gold and silver to costume jewelry. This is totally up to your taste and your budget.

In general, people use the tetragrammaton as a talisman for protection purposes, placing them on the door of their house to prevent the entry of bad entities or bad spirits. There are also those who carry it with them, either wearing it as a necklace or elsewhere on their bodies. The important thing is that, like any other talisman, you make sure to clean it from time to time, to ensure that it is in the best condition to function as protection against bad influences or spirits.

To consecrate your tetragrammaton, you will need:

A tetragrammaton
A lodestone or a magnet
A yellow fabric sachet (or a larger bag if your tetragrammaton is larger in size)
The seven abundance seeds: white rice, corn, black beans,
    lentils, chickpeas, pinto beans, and fava beans.
A bay laurel leaf for victory over evil.

On a Sunday, during the planetary hours of the sun, which you can find in the correspondence tables in the back of this book, touch your tetragrammaton with the lodestone while focusing on the virtues that you want this talisman to have. Then you are going to place the tetragrammaton, lodestone, the seeds, and the bay leaves inside of the yellow fabric bag. Repeat the following prayer:

> *I, (your name), consecrate you with the power of the creator*
> *by the virtues of the sun, by the powers of air, fire, water, and earth,*
> *so that by your powerful name I obtain divine protection, drive*
> *away all evil and ill intent against me, and return it to their ori-*
> *gins. Amen.*

Leave your tetragrammaton inside of the bag during the sun planetary hours. After that it is ready for its use.

La Herradura: The Horseshoe

The horseshoe is a magical symbol that is considered the oldest talisman in the world. This talisman has been used for centuries to ward off evil and bring good luck and fortune in Mexico. It is typically either worn as a necklace or hung above doors. This symbol protects the person or home's inhabitants from evil spirits, harmful witchcraft, and malevolent intent from others, while bringing blessings and attracting good business. This talisman is highly special. This would not be a Brujeria de Rancho book if I neglected to include the most powerful rancho talisman there is, *la herradura*.

Just like I told you in the beginning of this book, magic runs in both sides of my family. Even though both sides are magical, they each have their own ways to do magic. But there is a belief that they share that began in the time of the Mexican Revolution. It is said that whoever finds a horseshoe along their path should hold onto it with their left hand and make a wish out loud, then throw the horseshoe back behind them. They must then continue walking forward without looking to see where it has fallen.

Rancho's Horseshoe Consecration

For the consecration that my Grandma Socorro used to do, you will need:

> The horseshoe (either to hang above your door or a pendant to wear as a necklace)
> A lodestone or magnet
> Holy Water
> Cracked corn, flaked maize, or even corn meal (whatever you have available)
> Red string or ribbon
> New cleaning rags

On a Monday during the moon planetary hours, clean you horseshoe or horseshoe necklace with the new rag and Holy Water. After it's clean, touch your horseshoe with the lodestone or magnet with each hand and focus on your intention. (In this case, your intention is to ward off evil and bring good luck and fortune.) Follow these specific instructions: Grab the lodestone or magnet with the left hand first and, while touching the horseshoe, say, *"Protect me/us, ward me/us, extract from us illnesses and bad-spirited intentions thrown at me/us."*

Then grab the lodestone or magnet with the right hand and, again while touching the horseshoe with the lodestone or magnet, say, *"Bring me/us good opportunities, bring me/us good fortune, everything."*

Afterwards, place the horseshoe in a bowl and cover with the maize. Dip a clean rag in the Holy Water and lay it on top. Leave it there for the remainder of the planetary hour. Remove your horseshoe or necklace from the bowl and repeat the following popular prayer:

> *By the Holy Trinity, horseshoe, I entrust you in the name of the Father God, the Son, and the Holy Spirit, to bring (me/us) health, good luck, and money. Saint James, when you walked through the mountains, among thorns, thistles, and with many enemies behind you, that you later blindfolded, with your great power, I need that power. Just as you put a horseshoe on your horse, and that power within it, you got rid of the battlefield and your enemies, I need a little of that great power, that God has given to you, to be put into this horseshoe, so that it brings good opportunities, wealth, and happiness.*

> *By the name of the great Apostle James, this magnetized horseshoe will get (me/us) out of any unfortunate situation and bad places and circumstances without anyone knowing or noticing and remove everything meant to harm (me/us) and keep (me/us) safe from (my/our) enemies and fatal events. Get riches and honors and have all the people I want to love me. Free me from everything and save me from my enemies and any life-threatening situations that may occur. All this I believe as if I am seeing it through your incomparable virtues. I wish at this time that this magnet*

horseshoe, so powerful in itself, grants me these virtues and gifts.
All this I believe, and I entrust to Saint James to be fulfilled, and
the name of God, and this powerful horseshoe. Amen.

Hang the horseshoe above your door with the ends pointing up on an odd numbered day, preferably at night when the moon is out. It should be hung with a red string or ribbon. If you are consecrating a horseshoe necklace, it can also be worn on a metal chain.

The Fixed Horseshoe of Saint Martín of Tours

San Martín Caballero (Saint Martin the Horseman or Chevalier) is a folk name for Saint Martín of Tours, who is a very popular saint in Mexico. He is invoked by those in need for good luck, financial success, business improvement, or any endeavor that involves travel. He is the patron saint of shop owners, business, travelers, and soldiers. On the other hand, he is also popular amongst gamblers. This is because they believe that the horse he rides is related to the lucky horseshoe. He is certainly the epitome of good luck among the Mexican community. His feast day is celebrated on November 11.

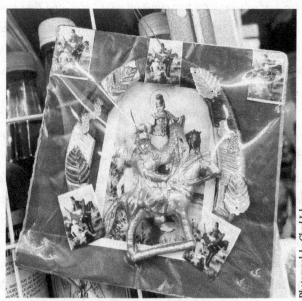

Photograph by Chad Johnson

Martín's parents were Pagan, but he discovered Christianity as a youth and converted at age ten, although he was not baptized. When he was fifteen years old, Martín, who was from a military family and in fact named after Mars, the Roman patron of war and soldiers, joined the Roman army, where he would later become the head of the Imperial Cavalry. One day he encountered a beggar in Amiens. The beggar was unclothed and very cold, so Martín removed his cloak and with his sword, he cut it in half. He gave half to the beggar and dressed himself in the remnant. That night, Martín had a vision in which Christ appeared to him. The vision spoke to him, "Martín, a mere catechumen has clothed me." A catechumen is one who is being instructed in the Christian faith and not yet baptized.

Unlike the tradition of my Grandmother Socorro, who dictated that a horseshoe must be hung with the ends in a vertical position, the horseshoes of my Grandmother Diana were hung with the ends pointing downwards and with the image of San Martín Caballero or another saint on a red fabric-lined frame inside of the horseshoe.

To consecrate this talisman that my Grandma Diana used to make, you will need:

A horseshoe
Holy Water
A new cleaning rag
A lodestone
A bowl
Seven ajo machos (if you cannot get ajo macho, you can use
garlic cloves, but traditionally ajo machos are used)
One package of lentils
Rosemary
Eleven coins of the highest accessible denomination circulating in your
country. Grandma used the 10 pesos ones. If you are in the United
States, use the dollar coin, you can get them in any bank.
An image of Saint Martín Caballero

On a Tuesday, during Mars planetary hours, clean the horseshoe with the cleaning rag and Holy Water. Once it is clean, place it in the bowl and cover it with the lentils, the lodestone, the rosemary, the seven ajo macho, and the eleven coins, and leave it there for the planetary hour. Remove the eleven coins from the bowl. Carry them with you and give them away to the first beggar you encounter asking for money. Lastly, take the horseshoe and the lodestone out of the bowl and say the appropriate prayer from among the following list, touching the horseshoe with the lodestone with your dominant hand while you do.

Horseshoe Prayer for Business:

> *Oh! Horseshoe of good fortune, I ask you, that in the name of San Martín Caballero, that the charity of his soul brings a lot of clients to this business. May his miraculous sword banish hexes, and the envy of my jealous competitors, and that you, horseshoe of his spirited steed, bring me luck in all my ideas, projects, and sales. Oh, Saint Martín Caballero! Of the faithful missionary Lord. Keep this business safe from all evil! Always protect it! So that it never misses good clients, money, and prosperity. Oh! Lucky horseshoe, give me your help so that my business never lacks this blessing. For being generous we venerate you, glorious Saint Martín Caballero, be forever praised and welcomed to my business. Amen.*

Horseshoe Prayer for Home:

> *Oh, glorious Roman soldier, that you were conferred by God to fulfill the will of charity, for the greatest trials that you underwent, I ask you with all my heart to fight every need in my house. May the horseshoe of your miraculous horse banish all sickness and danger and provide everyone living in here health, peace, food. Amen.*

Creating the Horseshoe Talisman

The materials needed to construct your horseshoe talisman in the tradition of my Grandma Diana can be found in most craft or hardware stores. You will need:

Consecrated horseshoe
Scissors
Ribbon (check the table in Chapter 14 for color correspondences)
A plywood square (6x6 inches)
Red fabric
Silicone glue gun
Silicone glue sticks
Staples
Fiber fill
Your favorite gold and silver charms
Glitter
Sequins of assorted colors
Glue (preferably strong all purpose clear glue)
Plastic wrap
Picture hanging wire
Hammer and nails
Saint Martin Caballero prayer card or image

Attach the fiber fill to the plywood using the glue gun. Place the red fabric over the fiber fill again, attaching it with the glue gun. Wrap your horseshoe with the ribbon; do not leave any of the metal exposed. Using the hammer and nail, punch holes in the plywood to both secure the horseshoe to the board and to be able to hang your talisman on the wall. Glue the San Martín prayer card or image to the center of the wood, then secure the horseshoe over top of the prayer card using the wire. Using the glue, decorate with the charms, glitter, or sequins to make your talisman your own and visually appealing to you. Once your glue is dry, wrap the entire talisman with plastic wrap to ensure none of the decorations come off. Insert the wire through the holes you made to hang the talisman.

Select your location over your front door, place a nail into the wall, and attach your talisman.

Ojo Turco: Nazar Eye

You may be wondering, how did we end up with the *nazar* eye in a book on Mexican sorcery? A nazar (from the Arabic word meaning sight or surveillance) is an ancient talisman in the shape of an eye that is believed to protect from the Evil Eye. It is a popular talisman in many cultures and traditions, including and especially among Jews. Among the Jews who emigrated to Mexico, many of them came from Turkey. These Jews spoke Ladino, a

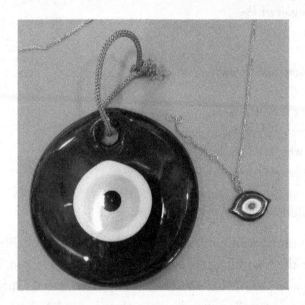

Spanish-Jewish dialect spoken by Sephardic Jews. (This language is also called Spaniolish.) The majority of these Jews ended up in Northeastern Mexico. The *ojo turco* (as it's called in Spanish) or nazar is traditionally made of glass, although other materials can be used. This talisman is hung in the home or worn on the body as jewelry in order to ward off and protect against the Evil Eye.

The Evil Eye, according to popular tradition, is a kind of negative energy given off by someone who envies or admire very intensely another person. This causes a deterioration in the target's mental and physical health. The Evil Eye does not have to be given intentionally, although it can be— sometimes the caster's subconscious desire is enough to manifest it. The most effective prevention method is the use of this talisman.

To consecrate this talisman, you will need:

A nazar eye
Red ribbon
Lodestone
Holy Water
A new rag
Rue
Three garlic cloves
A package of chickpea legumes.
A bowl

On a Tuesday, during Mars planetary hours, clean your nazar eye with the new rag and Holy Water. Place it in the bowl with the lodestone and add the chickpeas, garlic cloves, and rue. Cover it with the rag you used and leave it there during the planetary hour. Afterwards, take the nazar out of the bowl.

Pray the following prayer while touching the talisman with the lodestone held in your dominant hand:

> *Heavenly God! You who have been the verb made man, and grace, You who live in heaven, guiding and protecting us, I ask you to protect me, to keep me from all evil, from the diseases, the illnesses, and the bad fortune, that others' eyes throw at me in the form of the Evil Eye. Don't let anything touch my being, my soul, and my property because only you reside in them, that jealousy, adulation or flattery does not cause me the Evil Eye.*

Hamsa

The hamsa is a symbol that has had numerous other names throughout the age like the hand of Fatima and the hand of Miriam, and has been variously interpreted by scholars as a Jewish, Christian, Islamic, and even a Pagan talisman. Yet even as the magical form remains shrouded in mystery and scholars debate nearly every aspect of its emergence, it is recognized today as an important symbol in Mexican folk magic and art. It is difficult to pinpoint the exact time when hamsas emerged in Mexican culture, though it is clearly a symbol of Sephardic nature that is still very present in the Northeastern side of Mexico and South Texas. Today, you can get a hamsa in every botanica or artsy shop.

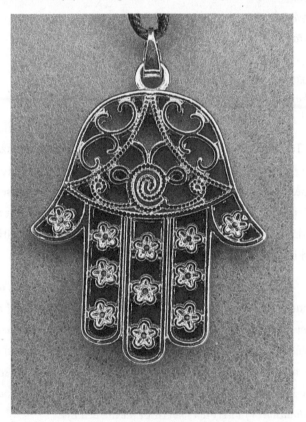

Many Mexicans have Crypto-Jewish ancestors who fled to the borderlands in order to escape death and persecution. There is a well-founded myth about the founder of the city of Monterrey, Nuevo León, and surroundings. It is said that Diego de Montemayor, vice regent to Luis Carvajal y de la Cueva, settled with twelve families to represent the twelve tribes of Israel with the idea of establishing a new land of the Jews. It is also believed that after the Jewish expulsion from Spain in 1492, exiled Jews used a Hamsa as protection in the foreign lands to which they were forced to relocate. When you combine these two stories, it's easy to see how the hamsa could have become such a powerful cultural symbol of protection in Mexico.

To consecrate your hamsa, you will need:

A hamsa
Five garlic cloves
Rue
Salt
Rosemary
Holy water
Cleaning rag
Lodestone
A bowl

On a Tuesday, during Mars planetary hours, clean your hamsa with Holy Water and then place it in your bowl. Add the five garlic cloves, rue, rosemary, salt, and the lodestone, and leave them in the bowl with the hamsa during Mars planetary hours. Afterwards, remove the hamsa and the lodestone from the bowl. Repeat one of the following prayers based on your needs while touching your hamsa with your lodestone, which should be held in your dominant hand.

If you plan to hang your hamsa in your home: *Let no sadness come through this gate. Let no trouble come to this dwelling. Let no fear come through this door. Let no conflict be in this place. Let this home be filled with the blessing of joy and peace.*

If you plan to wear your hamsa as jewelry: *Let no sadness come to this heart. Let no trouble come to these arms. Let no conflict come to these eyes. Let my soul be filled with the blessing of joy and peace.*

There are different versions of these prayers, and the text is commonly written in either Hebrew, English, or Spanish. It is believed that this folk prayer may have originated from a poem. Once you complete this step, your hamsa is ready.

All-Powerful Hand

Have you ever heard the terminology "powerful hand?" The *Mano Ponderosa* or All-Powerful Hand is a specifically Catholic incarnation of a Roman predecessor. It looks like a hand with five small figures atop the fingers: Baby Jesus on the thumb; Saint Joseph on the index finger; the Virgin Mary on the middle finger; Saint Joachim, Mary's father, on the ring finger; and Saint Anne, Mary's mother, on the pinkie.

In the folk magical customs of rural areas in Mexico, it is believed that whoever wears the Powerful Hand or hangs this image in their dwelling is protected against bad arts and witchcraft.

To consecrate the Powerful Hand, you will need:

A Powerful Hand medal or image (the Powerful Hand is
    hung in the home in a small picture frame)
Frankincense
Myrrh
Bay leaves
Vegetable charcoals
Matches
A charcoal resistant container

On a Tuesday, during Saturn planetary hours, burn the frankincense, myrrh, and bay leaves over the charcoal in your charcoal resistant container. Pass your Powerful Hand through the resulting smoke five times while you repeat the following prayer:

> *House of Jerusalem, where Jesus Christ entered, evil came*
> *out at the same time, leaving good at the same time. I ask Jesus of*
> *Nazareth, come into my home too. Get the evil out of here and keep*

the good for me. In the name of the Living God, Maria, Joseph, and the Powerful Hand. Amen.

Powerful Hand to Vanquish an Enemy

The Powerful Hand also has a sinister side. To vanquish an enemy and throw a malediction on them, you should, on a Tuesday or Friday, face the direction in which your enemy lives. Hold the Powerful Hand and focus on your enemy's downfall as you repeat in silence the following infamous prayer:

> Powerful Hand that provides me protection and blessings, I invoke you, here in this hour, in this moment, in this place. Make yourself present so that I can get rid of this enemy and all the ones that are plotting to cause me damage or hurt me, so everything is returned to them multiplied by five. If one has wished me death, I deliver this person to you, so, you, with no mercy, turn the light off the life of my enemy. And if my enemy wishes me ill in love matters, I ask that this person dies alone having never been loved. If this harm is wished upon me in money or business matters, I name you as my intercessor, my justice fighter, justice giver; you powerful sacred hand, make this person poor and with a bad name in much debt. Who goes against me, make such a person a loser, and that which my enemy has, make it my possession.
>
> Cut the tongue of whomever is dirtying my name and don't forget to bless who blesses my name and speaks highly about me. Protect me from witchcraft, misadventures, and demons. Guide me to me good fortune, health, money, and love. While my light shines in this earth, may my hand be held by your powerful hand. Amen.

This practice is often associated with brujas de rancho and old-fashioned brujeria.

CHAPTER FIVE

WORKING WITH SAINTS

"I am truly your merciful Mother, yours and all the people who live united in this land and all the other people of different ancestries, my lovers who love me, those who seek me, those who trust in me. Here I will hear their weeping, their complaints, and heal all their sorrows, hardships and sufferings."

—Our Lady of Guadalupe

Although it is true that Mexico is a predominantly Catholic country, Catholicism is not lived as in other places. In Mexico, whether you are a believer or not, saints are special, and most saints are venerated, beseeched, thanked, and given offerings.

I have always said that necessity opens the doors to magic, and magic opens the doors you want to be opened. There is a very famous quote: "Pobre México, tan lejos de Dios y tan cerca de Estados Unidos," which translates, "Poor Mexico, so far from God and so close to the United States." This quote was misattributed to former Mexican president Porfirio Díaz, however, it was written by the Nuevo León intellectual Nemesio García Naranjo. This quote caused quite a stir among the church and international politicians and diplomats but it summarizes how the average Mexican feels with precision.

This faith and full trust in the martyrs and saints was born from the extreme need of Mexicans. Many times we refer to saints as "our amulets" or as our buddies, pals, or intercessors due to the belief that they can resolve favors or problems for us before the "omnipotent" god, who, due to cultural issues and resentment, many feel is distant and out of reach.

For some people, our ways of exercising our faith in the saints may seem profane, even laughable because they are unaware of our heavy cultural baggage. For others, like me, these beliefs are magical. When the new religion was imposed on our ancestors, they had another vision. They accepted new prayers and practices because, in some way, they found a similarity with the one already theirs, keeping their culture deep in their hearts and thoughts. In this way, over time and over the years, our rituals and offerings managed to survive. Although they are not totally pure, they are strongly loaded in essence with the worship of our ancient gods. This phenomenon is called syncretism.

The personalities and backgrounds of the saints you encounter in this chapter are vibrant and nuanced. Some of these saints even have quite dark pasts or personality traits, attributed to popular folklore.

Working with Estampitas: Prayer Cards

In the Catholic tradition, holy cards or prayer cards are small devotional pictures. They usually depict a religious scene or a saint and are roughly the size of a playing card. The reverse side of the card typically contains a prayer. If you are in the United States and have ever been to a Catholic funeral, you have likely encountered prayer cards already; they are often distributed as part of the service. Prayer cards first appeared in the 1500s. These cards are very affordable; their value comes not from a monetary worth but from the devotional connection to the saint and the meaningful relationships they represent. You can find prayer cards for folk saints as well as saints canonized by the Church.

Prayer cards have several purposes in Mexican magic. They can serve as a lucky amulet, or they can be fixed to use as protection. In this chapter I also discuss some more infamous ways to use prayer cards.

Saint Expedite and Addictions in Mexico

Saint Expedite is the patron saint of people who need things in a hurry, those who are desperate and need something so fast that it could even be life or death. However, in Mexico, Expedite is also petitioned for relief of addiction, including recovery for alcoholics, gamblers, and drug addicts. It is very common to see people giving away Saint Expedite prayer cards outside of meetings such as Alcoholics Anonymous.

Saint Expedite is traditionally depicted holding a cross with the word *Hodie*, "today" in Latin, written on it. His foot is stepping on a crow, which is portrayed uttering the word *Cras*, Latin for "tomorrow." In this way Saint Expedite is depicted as putting his foot down on "doing it later" in favor of "doing it today."

In Mexico, Alcoholics Anonymous and Narcotics Anonymous have a powerful method that allows addicts to move forward and overcome obstacles: doing something *solo por hoy* or "just for today." The philosophy of living life "just for today" is why a lot of people started asking Saint Expedite for recovery for themselves or their family members and why Saint Expedite prayer cards are given away as a way of testimony.

Saint Expedite and I have our own story, a long and sad one that began when I was a child. When we grow up in a household with addiction problems, we develop other addictions that are much sneakier and more nefarious as a coping mechanism. We might not even notice these addictions exist. An addiction is essentially a ritual that prevents us from living a productive life and taking care of our needs—a ritual that causes destruction in our lives in some way.

Codependency is an emotional and behavioral condition that affects an individual's ability to have a healthy, mutually satisfying relationship. To put it simply, codependency means being addicted to another person or to a relationship. Codependency is the absence of a relationship with self. This cycle can occur in romantic relationships, friendships, parent-child relationships, and many other relationship dynamics where the "giver" tends to be overly responsible, making excuses for the "taker" and assuming responsibility over their obligations. Givers are self-critical and often perfectionistic. Fixing or rescuing others makes them feel needed.

I was so busy and prompt to fix, ask, go, resolve, make up for, that I was focusing on other people's addictions. Meanwhile, mine was way more severe and out of control. I wish I would have known before what I know today, that enabling as a behavior is part of co-dependence, helping another person in a way that allows their addiction to continue with no consequences. Negative enabling hurts everybody. It prevents growth in the person who is enabled and creates resentment in the enabler. I crippled a lot of people, I enabled them with my magic, with my actions, with everything that I have and didn't have. What if instead of asking Saint Expedite for their recovery, I had asked for mine?

If we can't hold ourselves accountable, we can't hold other people accountable. My beef with Saint Expedite lasted many years, but today it is over. I didn't understand at the time that in his infinite mercy he did not bail me out with that petition, otherwise I wouldn't be here in the US or writing a book for the community. I can say that at the time that was by far my worst blow out, and I never gave it thought until today.

Ritual to Make Someone Hate Alcohol

This is an ancient Mexican ritual that Mexican women performed to help their alcoholic husbands or kids with addiction. Viewed with a 2022 lens, everybody should be responsible for their addictions, seek professional help, go to meetings, get therapy, and in some cases be prescribed psychiatric medication to fight alcoholism. Every case is different and this spell should not be used as a replacement for other types of addiction help and counseling. Take care of yourself and do your research. If you are struggling, seek help for yourself as well!

I have seen this ritual work but it is very aggressive. Usually, the alcoholic starts to develop some kind of "weird" allergy to alcohol. Symptoms I have seen include rashes, vomiting, and headaches. It's not that the target of this ritual doesn't crave it anymore, it's that they can't consume it without punishment.

You will need:

A photograph of the alcoholic person.
A glass bottle with lid
Lemon juice concentrate
Holy Water
A small piece of cotton
Drink consumed by the alcoholic
Scotch tape
Saint Expedite prayer card
Permanent marker

Take the bottle and fill it halfway with the lemon juice concentrate. Fill the other half with the drink the person is consuming. Place the photograph inside the bottle. While inserting the photo, repeat: *May this vice become sour and bitter in (person's pronouns) mouth along with a horrible rash every time (person's pronouns) tongue touches a single drop of alcohol.*

At that moment, you will visualize the person becoming tired of the vice, overcoming their addiction, fighting, and progressing. Close and seal the bottle with tape. Before finishing the ritual, wet a small piece of cotton with Holy Water and clean the entire outside of the bottle with it, then tape the Saint Expedite prayer card to the bottle. Write cras (tomorrow) on the bottom, and on the top draw a cross with the word hodie (today) written on it. Let them touch the bottom of the bottle. (Every time the addict relapsed, the grandmothers touched the bottom of that bottle and tapped seven times along with saying seven Hail Marys.) Afterwards, keep it in a secret place, out of reach of the person with the problem in question.

When seven months have passed, repeat the ritual again. Take the old bottle out of the house and spill out the contents. Once it is empty, you must set it on fire to burn all the bad vibrations it has absorbed.

To Find a Desired Job

Santa Clara of Assisi is a very miraculous saint. We can turn to her when we cannot find a way out of some daily situations. The main reason why we work with her in our search for employment is because she performed miracles to multiply loaves of bread, and bottles of oil appeared in her convent where were none before. This hechizo with this noble saint will help you to get a job and ensure that there is no lack of the daily bread on the table.

You will need:

An image or prayer card of Santa Clara
One glass of water
Your spell scissors
One piece of white unlined paper (plain printer paper works well)
Your personal perfume
One white candle

On your completely blank, unlined paper that you cut into a square with your spell scissors, write your name and date of birth three times. Bless yourself three times in the name of the Father, the Son, and the Holy Spirit, asking Santa Clara that, with this offering you place for her, your supplication will be answered. Place the paper inside the glass right side up so that the letter can be seen. Place three touches of your personal perfume in the glass, then fill the glass with water up to the middle point. Place the prayer card or image and the candle behind the glass of water. Ask Santa Clara to find the job you need soon. If you already have a specific employer that you desire, then ask Santa Clara that you will soon receive a call from that place. When that happens, go to the interview with the same prayer card or image in your wallet.

To Overcome Financial Violence

La burra no era arisca, la hicieron a palos. (The mule wasn't ill-tempered, they made her so by beating her with sticks.)

Mexico has one of the highest rates of gender violence in the world. To put the scale of this into context is difficult because it is so engrained in our culture and has been for generations. A lot of us don't have an idea of what our grandmas put up with in their lives. This culture of abuse is endemic: many women in the US and other countries are struggling with centuries of machismo, misogyny, and forms of insidious abuse.

Abusive partners use physical, sexual, emotional, and economic tactics in order to isolate, diminish, control, exploit, and terrorize their partners. Economic abuse is defined as controlling a woman's ability to acquire, use, and maintain economic resources. Women with abusive partners often face serious threats to their financial wellbeing and barriers toward realizing their personal financial capability.

In Mexico, financial violence is so normalized that it is often difficult to detect. There is a classic Mexican song called "Oye Bartola" that, when viewed from today's lens, is a horrific example of what financial violence can look like in some cases. The lyrics tell a story of a man "giving" a woman all the "control" of financial decisions for the family, only to turn around and criticize her decisions, painting her as having unrealistic understanding of what things cost. Other examples of financial violence include controlling paychecks and bank accounts, preventing a woman from accessing transportation or using isolation tactics to prevent her from working, and perpetrating violence against women and children by withholding and dodging child support and other payments.

To take control and make someone who is abusing you financially give you your money, you will need:

One coin of the highest denomination in your country. The coin must come out of your partner's money and your partner must hand it to you. If the spell is to reinforce child support, the child must receive it into their hands.
Red yarn or thread
One Mano Ponderosa prayer card
One white candle or, for an extra kick, a cordero manso candle
A permanent marker

Write the full name and date of birth of the person you want to dominate economically on the back of the prayer card. Light the candle. Take the coin and hold it in the candle flame, burning it on all sides as you say the following: This is the money in the hands of (name of the person to dominate), so that just as this coin is burned, so are your hands feeling burned until you give me (or your children) your money.

Persinate (make the sign of the cross) and say three Hail Marys. After heating the coin, place it above your powerful hand and wrap it with the red cord until it is completely covered while saying these words:

> *This is not a coin, it is the hands of (person's name), so that*
> *just as I tie this coin, I tie your hands and your money to my will so*
> *that you give it to me (or my children). So be it.*

Bless yourself with the coin and place the prayer card together with the coin in your bra (or pocket) for three days.

Saint Hedwig: To Help Build Credit and Repay Debt

You will need:

One white candle
A prayer card or image of Saint Hedwig
Rosemary
Olive oil
Vinegar
A glass of water
White paper
Scissors
Black pen
Clay plate

On the paper, write the amount of money owed and the name of every debtor. Anoint the candle with the olive oil and rosemary. Place the paper under the plate. Light the candle and after the candle is burnt out, place the paper on top of the plate. Pour the vinegar over top of it until you can no longer read the writing. While you are doing this, recite the following prayer:

> O glorious Saint Hedwig, you who were and are the shelter of the poor and the aid of the indebted, and who today receive the eternal blessing from the Lord, today I ask you to be my intercessor so that I can respect my financial commitments and clear my name of all debt and all unfinished business and transactions. Glorious Saint Hedwig help and intercede for me I pray to you, so I can find financial freedom. Amen.

Saint Martin de Porres: Protection for Hate, Intolerance, and Discrimination

Hate, intolerance, and discrimination often manifest as an unwillingness to accept and respect views, beliefs, choices, or behavior that differs from one's own viewpoints. Intolerance and its terrible effects unfortunately are pretty much a day-to-day thing for Brujeria de Rancho practitioners and our people, so how do we protect ourselves?

If you feel you are a target for intolerance and discrimination for any reason, carry with you a miniature broom wrapped with a one-decade wooden rosary along with a Saint Martin de Porres prayer card.

Saint Martin de Porres, the Holy Man of the Broom, is one of the most important Brujeria de Rancho spirits we work with, due to the closeness to the practitioners and the struggles we deal with on a daily basis as mestizos and immigrants. Martin was born in Lima, Peru in 1579, the son of a Spanish knight, Don Juan de Porres, and the former Panamanian slave Ana Velazquez. His father initially refused to acknowledge the boy publicly as his own, because Martin, like his mother, was Black. Though Martin's father later helped to provide for his education, his son faced difficulties because of his family background.

Martin's spiritual practices were legendary. Equally legendary were his love of animals and his powers, which included visions, ecstasies, healing, supernatural understanding, and bilocation, a practice by which one person can appear in two separate physical locations at the same time. Some of his peers said they encountered him in places as far off as Japan even as he remained in Lima. While he faced discrimination, Martin's kindness, his love of prayer, and humility helped him become friends with many people from all social classes, which enabled him to alleviate the sufferings of many. He died at age fifty-nine on November 3rd, 1639 and was canonized by Pope Saint John XXIII on May 6, 1962. His feast day is celebrated every November 3rd.

Prayer to Saint Martin de Porres

This prayer can be personalized and tailored to the individual person based on their protection needs. Focus on the areas of your life where you face discrimination and pray the following to Saint Martin de Porres.

> *San Martín de Porres, my dear friend, there are many who reject my life, the way that I live it, the color of my skin, my religion, my sexual orientation, my socioeconomic class, my immigration status. I ask you to revive my love and trust in myself, and for you to touch the hearts of those who misjudge me and cause me harm. San Martin, friend of mine, you who knows the wounds of my history, the rejections, limitations, and the attacks that I have suffered. Make these people understand that they make a mistake and, with your holy broom, sweep all hatred from their heart and souls, but in case their souls and hearts are so dirty and impossible to clean, sweep them away from the path that I walk. Amen.*

Working with Saint Martin
de Tours to Bring Clientele

It's important to remember that devotion to the saints involves knowing about their lives and following their example. For example, shop owners must also commit to following San Martin's path. My parents, for example, had a clothing store, so I know that managing your business and making a profit while simultaneously modeling San Martin's generosity can be difficult. San Martin notably received a vision of Jesus Christ after he cut his own cloak to give half to an unclothed beggar. Following San Martin's example doesn't mean giving away your merchandise for free—your business would collapse. But if you serve with kindness, patience, and fair prices, among other virtues, you are giving everything you can and your clients will feel grateful for your service. My parents used to put on a big sale called 11/11, in honor of San Martin's feast day, so that people with low incomes could benefit from that bargain and purchase affordable winter clothing for their kids. You could do something similar. Be creative in your kindness!

For this spell to bring in clientele, you will need:

An image of San Martín Caballero.
A San Martin candle or red candle
Hay, pastor grass, or an apple (anything that would feed a horse)
A bowl filled with water
A handful of raw rice

This spell can be done on a Tuesday or another day of your preference. You can do it today! Place the image of the saint somewhere you feel comfortable, either on an altar or elsewhere. Fill the bowl with water. Place the water bowl next to the horse feed (the hay, pastor grass, or apple) in front of San Martin's image. Be plentiful and generous with the feed. Throw a little rice at the image of San Martin's feet and say the following:

As I give you this rice, I need your intercession to turn these
grains into money, prosperity, material abundance, and attract

good customers to my business. I am also feeding your horse to help
you bring me, quickly, a lot of clients, and good business, so be it!

Change the water and the horse feed while praying to Saint Martin on Tuesdays.

To Cut Witchcraft Against Your Business

You can ask Saint Martin Caballero for help in a desperate situation where you and your business are a target of witchcraft or salación. This prayer is to be prayed for seven Tuesdays in a row to neutralize a spell or curse when one's business is under a malediction.

You will need:

A San Martin Caballero seven-day candle
Holy water
Seven ajo machos

On every Tuesday for seven successive weeks, hide an ajo macho in your business place. Afterwards, light your candle and repeat the following prayer:

O glorious Roman soldier, who was of God conferred to ful-
fill the gift of charity! Because of the greatest trials to which you
were subjected by the Lord, I ask you with all my heart that you
fight the curses, witchcraft, and maledictions the envious sent to
my business, that the charity of your soul follow me wherever I
go. May your miraculous sword banish the curses in my life and
may the horseshoes of your spirited steed bring me luck in all my
dealings. Oh, Saint Martin Caballero of the faithful missionary
Lord, deliver me from all evil! Always protect me so that I never lack
health, work, and sustainment! Amen.

On the seventh Tuesday, let the whole candle be consumed. (Do not let it burn all the way down prior to this Tuesday.) On the eighth Tuesday, remove the ajos. Dispose of them carefully far away from your business.

Saint Elena's Nails: Dominate Feelings and Make Someone Love You

If you want to dominate a person and make them love you, you need to go to Saint Elena. For a long time, Mexican brujos have asked her, through the use of her miraculous nails, to bring them someone's love or return a wayward lover. Saint Elena was the mother of Emperor Constantine, the first Christian emperor of Rome. An early convert to Christianity, it was said that she discovered the Holy Cross and the nails that were used in the Crucifixion of Jesus during her pilgrimage to the Holy Land. As legend has it, one of those nails was dedicated to preserve the throbbing pain of anguish, and the other to inflict it.

To make someone despair and love you, you will need:

A picture of your target
Red candle
Three gold-colored nails
Olive oil
Dried hibiscus
Cinnamon
A plate

On a Friday, place the picture of your target under the plate. Dress your candle with the olive oil, the hibiscus, and the cinnamon while you anoint your intention as well. Arrange the candle in the center of the plate (it must stand by itself) and place the nails to the right. Light the candle and pray the following prayer:

Glorious Saint Helena, daughter of the Queen of Jerusalem.
You went to Jerusalem, three nails you brought. You consecrated
the first one, and on Tuesday you threw it out to sea. The second
you gave to your brother, Cipriano, so that in battle he overcame
beforehand. I ask you for a loan and not a gift, the one that is still in
your blessed palm, to stick it in the soul of (person's name) so it does

not forget me, to sink it into (person's name) forehead so it keeps me
on its mind, to bury it in (person's name) heart. Saint Caralampio,
draw it to me. Saint Helena, the nail that I ask of you is to drill it
into (person's name) mind, so that (person's name) always thinks
of me. There will be no tranquility until you, (person's name),
come to me, loving, faithful, meek as a lamb, hot like a switch.
Tranquility will not come until you are exhausted and humiliated
at my feet and begging for my love.

Let the candle be fully consumed. Once it is consumed throw one of the nails into a river or the sea. Give away the second one to someone you would like to protect; they should use it as an amulet. Wrap the third nail in your underwear with the picture of your target and put it in a safe place.

Saint Sylvester Prayer

Saint Sylvester was pope when Christianity became the official religion of the Roman Empire. His feast day falls on December 31st. Since *Silvester Abend*, or "Sylvester's Eve," is also New Year's Eve, many Mexicans hold late-night parties. My grandmother and a lot of Mexican abuelas prayed to San Silvestre for protection from other brujas and ill or evil intent. For his fight in the defense of the interests of the Church, San Silvestre has an invocation to intercede in the defense of private property, as there is a strong belief in his power to prevent theft and offer protection from those who intend to damage or steal our material blessings.

If you suspect that a witch is trying to harm you or your family, or if you live in an unsafe neighborhood and want to protect your property, New Year's Eve is the perfect day to petition Saint Sylvester. You do not need to light a candle or conduct a special ritual; just pray the following prayer with faith and then hang a copy of it above your door.

Mighty Saint Sylvester, I beg you to break and finish with
all witchcraft, curse, spell, and any power related to it, that your

immense power ends and removes the witches who are exercising the power of darkness. Oh Saint Sylvester! Drive away and break the witch's spells, break the power of voodoo, hexes, potions, or any witchcraft that they have done to me or my family. Put me in a protective shield to be able to receive in my life peace, love, health, opportunities, and family unity. Deliver me from every witch and sorcerer in the name of Jesus our Lord. Amen.

San Antonio: To Find a Spouse

The feast of San Antonio (Saint Anthony of Padua) is celebrated on June 13th. This saint is considered the patron saint of marriages. In Mexican folk magic, he is entrusted with the petitions for marriage and serious intentions. The saint is offered thirteen special coins of any denomination glued on a red ribbon on the day of his patronal feast.

This ritual has been successfully celebrated for centuries in Mexico. These coins are not going to be so easy to get, since they must be given to you by thirteen widows, who after being widowed have never "sinned" again (in other words, have sex again after being widowed). That is the original tradition.

A couple friends of mine in the US altered this tradition and instead asked thirteen "marriage material" people (essentially, the kind of person that they would like to be married to) to gift them the coins. This gave them amazing results! As I write these words, I'm getting ready to go to a wedding in Wisconsin of a friend of mine who followed this spell.

You can offer the ribbon at your church or on your altar. The requirements to invoke Saint Anthony are simple: It is required to build a home altar in a quiet place in the house and place his image on a white tablecloth. Offer white flowers, which are a symbol of purity, and white candles. The best incense to offer would be crafted from lilies. Saint Anthony is invoked on Fridays. The popular belief says that if a prudent time has passed without obtaining results, San Antonio should be turned upside down until he fulfills the task. It is known that Saint Anthony was very devoted to the Virgin Mary and the Child Jesus, therefore one of the best promises to make him in exchange for a favor is to pray the Holy Rosary for nine days and offer this novena in his name.

San Pancras and Parsley: To Attract Good Things in Life

Saint Pancras is the patron saint of children, jobs, shop owners, and health. I would not be writing this book without his intercession. Saint Pancras's feast is May 12th. It is customary to request favors from him by placing parsley beside his image. My grandma had a huge devotion for this saint. She had a big statue of him and every time she left the house, she used to rub the book Saint Pancras holds, while in his left hand he also holds a palm branch. On San Pancras' book are written the words *Venite Ad Me Et Dabo Vobis Omnia Bona*, which means "all good things come to me and I shall give them to you." While the Catholic Church views this as an invitation from the Gospel to trust in Jesus Christ, we in Brujeria de Rancho are way more literal and straightforward. This is how we work blessings from this saint.

You will need:

A Saint Pancras prayer card or statue
A glass 3/4 full of water
Fresh parsley
Dried parsley
Red ribbon
Seven pennies
One chunk of piloncillo (enough to fit comfortably in the water glass)
Green candle
Olive oil

On a Wednesday, fill a clear glass 3/4 of the way full with water. Tie your fresh parsley with the red ribbon. Add one chunk of piloncillo to the water. Dress your candle with the olive oil and dried parsley while you also anoint your intention. Add the seven pennies one by one to the glass; pray the Lord's Prayer for each penny you add. Once you finish, place the fresh parsley inside the glass and light the candle. Let the candle be consumed.

After the candle has burned down, remove the pennies from the glass and keep them with the statue or prayer card. Offer San Pancras fresh parsley every Wednesday. Rub his book every time you have a petition for him.

To Ask Saint Charbel for a Miracle

If you are facing a difficulty and need a miracle, do not hesitate to invoke Saint Charbel. He was introduced to Mexico in the early 1900s by Lebanese Maronite immigrants, and he has achieved an astounding popularity across the country. It is customary to place on his arms a ribbon in a color that corresponds to your petition. After the problem is resolved, a white ribbon with a thank you note must be added. When you walk into a church, his statue is covered with different colored ribbons for all of the favors that have been asked. You can hardly see the statue because of all the ribbons. It's a wonderfully colorful sight.

You will need:

Two ribbons, one white and the other one according to your petition
   (check the correspondences table at the back of this book)
A permanent marker

Repeat the following prayer: *Almighty God, who has manifested the power of Saint Charbel's intercession through his countless miracles and favors, grant us ...* (Here, state your intention and write it on the colored ribbon.) *... through his intercession. Amen.*

Place that ribbon on a Saint Charbel statue on his right side. This can be done either at your home altar or in a church. Once the petition is given, place the white ribbon with a thank you written on it on his left side.

Saint Cucuphas's Testicles:
To Find Something Lost

In some parts of Spain and Northeastern Mexico, we turn to Saint Cucuphas to help us find what has been lost. Saint Cucuphas is one of the most powerful saints to whom we can turn in these moments of real anguish. His name is reputedly of Phoenician origin and means "he who likes to joke." If you have misplaced something and cannot find it, it is customary to tie up the corner of a white handkerchief in a knot. If you *really* need to recover the lost item, you can tie up several corners and then repeat the following folk prayer to Saint Cucuphas every time you tie a knot: *"Saint Cucuphas, I'm tying your testicles in a knot and won't release them until I find what was lost."*

Do not forget to untie the knots once you have recovered your item.

San Marcos de Leon to Dominate and Tame

Prayers and conjures to Saint Marcos de Leon are very traditional in Mexican magic. The two main purposes of these prayers, conjures, and works through San Marcos de Leon are to dominate someone or tame someone. These prayers can be invoked not only for love relationships (the most common when it comes to domination and taming spells) but also for enemies or simply people in whom we need to exert a sense of calm and ease. If you are doing this domination spell for someone besides a romantic partner, modify the wording of the prayer below to best suit your purposes.

There is a legend that describes San Marcos de Leon (also known as Saint Mark) being thrown to the lions, only to have them neglect to attack him, outright refusing to do him any harm. The usually aggressive lions ended up sleeping at his feet while San Marcos de Leon gently caressed them.

In depictions of San Marcos in prayer cards, we often find him holding the Bible and writing. Often he is accompanied by a winged lion. To dominate the feelings of someone like San Marcos dominated the lions, you will need:

A San Marcos de Leon seven-day candle or an orange candle
Four cloves
A picture of your target
A Mexican clay plate

On a Friday night, take the picture of your target and place it on a surface facing downwards. Place the clay plate on top of the picture. Place the candle on top of the plate. Stick the four cloves into the candle in the form of a cross. Light the candle and repeat the following prayer:

> *Powerful San Marcos de León, you who have the power to tame beasts and dragons, I ask you to also tame the spirit of the person I love (say the name of the loved one), so that (person's pronouns) is dominated, and becomes docile with me. Powerful San Marcos de León, you who have the power to tame lions, I ask that the person I love (person's name) has good thoughts only toward me. San Marcos de León, I ask that the person I love (person's name) follow me, just as the living follow the cross and as the dead should follow the light. For your blessing, I ask San Marcos de León that you send my prayer to the Lord, so (person's name) body, mind, and spirit continues under my dominion and does my will. Amen.*

CHAPTER SIX

ENSALMOS AND REMEDIES

Take control of what I say, O LORD, and guard my lips.

Psalm 141:3

Ensalmos

Brujos de rancho live in a dual world where we walk through every side of the spectrum of the spiritual realm, which gives us the ability to perform wonderful and successful cleansings. Many brujos from the rancho are descendants of powerful and gifted *ensalmadores*.

Ensalmacion is the name of a folk healing practice that is practiced by some people who have a *don* (gift) to heal spiritual illnesses and afflictions with the use of tinctures and sacred prayers, requesting holy protection and relief for the bewitched one. Ensalmo is a very ancient method in Mexico, known to have esoteric, mystical, and magical powers. The person who performs it must be someone who possesses the virtue and the gift to impart it. The name *ensalmo* is taken from the Biblical psalms, as it is stated that as *ensalmeros* we usually use verses from the Psalter. The ensalmeros repeat these sacred prayers on certain days and at certain times to cure wounds, sores, or *apostemas* (blisters). In some cases, the ensalmo requires solutions such as alcohol or *agua del carmen* to disinfect and remove the affliction, in other cases cross-shaped scissors are placed on or passed over the patient's body. The *ensalmador* is a specialist in healing with words, and they are also hired to follow a coffin to pray and *dirige* (direct) a funeral from memory. Ensalmeros don't just pray, they pray *hard*; we know how to contact the spirit through those prayers.

Ensalmo practice was condemned by the Holy Inquisition in Mexico. There is a solid and large set of ensalmos that were documented by the Inquisition in the 1600s. These ensalmos await rescue and study, but as of the time of this writing that information remains only on those pages. The only other way to access it is through the oral tradition passed down to some brujos de rancho.

Ensalmos focus on the healing of spiritual illnesses such as Evil Eye and witchcraft. If we are unable to treat a certain condition, we must refer the patient to the right folk healer. Remember that these are healings for spiritual illnesses; this advice is not meant to replace that of a doctor or medical professional. An ensalmo requires a diagnosis. Brujos de rancho can diagnose it in different ways, by use of divination methods and the reading of the body. Digging into the patient's story and the ailment's symptoms allows us to identify patterns so we can make more effective decisions based on the patient's specific needs. This is why it is important for ensalmeros to understand and have a good working knowledge of other practices and that they are able to make good and on-time referrals as well.

The ensalmos that I am offering to you in this chapter are very traditional and ancient methods which have been performed successfully by brujas de rancho for centuries in our communities. For healing and relief, brujos de rancho crafted their own concoctions. Many of these had a base of cane alcohol, tequila, mezcal, raicilla, bacanora, sotol, aguardiente, or pulque mixed with different plants and herbs. These concoctions have the power to cure the Evil Eye, muscle aches, mosquito bites and different afflictions. When my legs ached, my grandmother rubbed them with peyote-infused alcohol.

Ensalmo to Cut the Evil Eye

The belief in the Evil Eye is far reaching and ancient, existing in many cultures, and Mexico is no different. Receiving the Evil Eye, which can be cast both voluntarily and involuntarily even through something as seemingly innocuous as an envious look, results in misfortune or illness. Babies are affected most frequently, but grown-up people can suffer from this as well.

For this ensalmo, you will need:

Sotol (or any distilled alcohol, such as what you would find for first aid use)
Rosemary
Sweet basil
Oregano
A metal or glass bottle (at least 7 oz.)
A small container

Pour 7oz of sotol (you can use other agave spirits or distilled alcohol) into your metal or glass bottle. Add a handful each of rosemary, sweet basil, and oregano. Let this mixture rest for at least nine days.

Once you have completed your preparation, the patient must step forward in front of your home altar. Put a little bit of your Evil Eye formula in a small container, so that you do not contaminate the whole mixture. I usually use a soda cap. Dip your spirit finger (ring finger) into the mixture and draw a cross on the patient's forehead. Repeat the following ensalmo:

> *In the name of the Father, the Son, and the Holy Spirit. (Say the name of the afflicted person), creature of God, I heal and ensalmo you from the Evil Eye, from the Evil Eye of witches and sorcerers, from the magnetic and demon-possessed stares, from hexes and imposed evils, and from any ailment that you have in your body, cutting it and destroying it, so it does not harm anyone. Jesus died on the cross and by the power of the cross I heal you, with these holy words and truths that are served to cut the evil that you (name of the afflicted person) have in your body.*

If it entered you through your feet and hands, Saint Amarus will cut and take it away from you; if it was through your heart, the Blessed Mother of God; if it was through the stomach, Saint Gregory; if by the throat, Saint Blaise; if by the belly, Saint Dominic; if by the mouth, Saint Raymond; if by the nose, Saint Beatriz; if by the eyes, Saint Lucy; if for the body, Saint Sebastian; if for the skin, Saint Roch; if by the front, Saint Vincent; if by the head, Saint John the Baptist; if for the joints, Saint Philip Nery; if it was from a dog bite, Saint Martin will cut its rage; if it is from an evil sorceress, Saint Lazarus will do this cut; if it is behind your back, our Lord Jesus Christ will cut it, since He is the one who can cut everything.

The three had promise, the three will cut it off from you, who are Father, Son, and Holy Spirit. Amen.

Ensalmo to Get Rid of Bad Shadows

This ensalmo is to get rid of bad shadows, also known as spirit attachments, or spiritual workings and hexes worked against us through cemetery spirits.

You will need:

Sotol (or any alcohol)
Bay leaf
Rosemary
Three cloves
A metal or glass bottle (at least 7 oz.)

In a metal or glass bottle, add 7 oz. of sotol (or other distilled alcohol) and a handful of crushed bay leaves, rosemary, and the three cloves. Let the mixture sit for nine days. Once this preparation is complete, the patient must step in front of your home altar. Put a small amount of the mixture in a small container so that you do not contaminate the whole bottle. I usually use a soda cap. Dip your spirit finger (ring finger) into the mixture and draw a cross on the patient's forehead. Repeat Saint Luis Beltran's Ensalmo.

In the name of the Father, the Son, and the Holy Ghost, I clean, I heal, and I banish from this body this afflicted cemetery spirit. In the name of the Holy Trinity, Father, Son, and Holy Spirit, three different people and their true virtue, and of the Virgin Mary, Our Lady, conceived without the stain of original sin, virgin before childbirth, in childbirth, and after delivery, and for the glorious Saint Gertrude, the eleven thousand virgins, Saint Joseph, Saint Roch, and Saint Sebastian, and for all the saints, angels, and archangels, for your glorious Incarnation, glorious Birth, Most Holy Passion, glorious resurrection, and Ascension. For the so high and Most Holy Mysteries that I firmly believe are my helpers in this task, I beg your Divine Majesty, to be my intercessor, and to the Blessed Mother and our advocate, to free and heal (name of the person) of this bad shadow spirit of the cemetery that is tormenting (person's pronouns) and causing (person's pronouns) harm. In all good faith I beseech you Lord, for your honor, and the devotion of those present, to serve you, and for your holiness and your mercy, heal and free (name of the person) of the ills and diseases that (person's pronouns) suffers, from this evil, this wound, sore or pain, mood or illness, taking them off from this body, and do not allow, your Divine Majesty, bad shadows, corruption, or any damage, overtake it again. I'm giving you full power over this body and this soul to heal them so that this creature can serve you and do your most holy will. Creature of God: I cleaned and healed you from all bad shadows and Jesus Christ Our Lord Redeemer healed and blessed you. Amen.

Ensalmo to Get Rid of Bad Air

Mal aire, or bad air, is one of the most famous and common diseases since pre-Hispanic times in Mexico. In pre-Hispanic beliefs, the "bad air" is acquired for several reasons. It could be that the affected person breathed directly from the breath of the water or rain gods, that a wind hit and entered the body of an overheated person, that the person breathed cemetery air that emanated from corpses or phantoms or from a place where a tragedy occurred, or that a brujo has sent the mal aire to their victim.

For this ensalmo to rid a person of mal aire, you will need:

Sotol or other distilled spirit or alcohol
Rue
Basil
Rosemary
A metal or glass bottle (at least 7 oz.)

In a metal or glass bottle, add 7 oz. of sotol (or other distilled spirit or alcohol), and a handful each of rue, basil, and rosemary. Let the mixture sit for nine days. Once you have completed your preparation, the patient must step in front of an altar. Put a little bit of your mixture into a small container so as not to contaminate the whole mixture. I usually use a soda cap. Dip your spirit finger (ring finger) into the mixture and draw a cross on the patient's forehead. Repeat the following Saint Michael's Ensalmo:

> *In the name of the Lord Almighty, through the action of the Archangel Michael, may all negativity within be removed, may the bad air be stripped of this body, and may all the symptoms of this spiritual evil disappear, as well as ties, obstacles, sickness, and aches, so be it in the name of the Almighty, through the power of Saint Michael. Amen.*

Repeat the prayer three times.

Rancho Esoteric Soaps

The primary reason why we use soap is to cleanse our body of dirt and feel refreshed again. There are some soaps that provide both physical and spiritual body cleansing and healing when used. Despite being made from the same natural ingredients found around us, such as plants and essential oils, some classic Mexican soaps are very magical and powerful. They are usually used as a purifying medium for personal use, ritual objects, or a selected space; however, they can also have an influence on issues such as love, prosperity, and health, among others. Brujas in the rancho are super specific about brands, not only for the quality but also for their prices. Grisi brand soaps are a classic for magical soaps. Grisi is a 100% Mexican pharmaceutical company that manufactures and markets leading products of natural origin, following the same formulas introduced since the company was founded in 1863.

How to Use Magical Soaps

First, preform a tolerance check to make sure that your skin does not have an adverse reaction your chosen soap. Rub a little bit of the soap on the inside of your arm and wait twenty-four hours to make sure there is no irritation. If your skin passes the tolerance check, you're good to go, but otherwise you should look for an alternative soap.

Prepare your soap by writing your intentions on it with a toothpick. As you write, pray three Hail Marys. Afterwards, leave them in velacion (candlelight) until the candle has been totally consumed. Now your magical soap is ready to use.

Brujas de rancho use soap for many different purposes, but a principal one is carving. Soaps are molded into the shapes of people, animals, or objects. The thought process behind soap carving is similar in fashion to a doll or a poppet—calling upon sympathetic magic to achieve an end. A soap carving in the likeness of a specific person is great for focusing your intention on that individual. I'm not as crafty as my grandma was, so I use a gingerbread man cookie cutter, and if I'm making a soap figure of a woman, I make the waist thinner and the hips more prominent. It's also common to carve names, birth dates, and other important information on the soap to bond it with the intended target. Carvings in the shape of a penis or vagina are also popular and have been successfully used for spells of sexuality and revenge.

Here is a list of the most popular soaps and their purposes. These soaps have been used for generations in Mexican folk magic.

Aloe vera soap: Aloe vera soap prevents accidents, drives away evil, and protects the user from negative entities and attachments. It is highly recommended to use before and after going to the cemetery. It keeps skin moist and fresh, and helps sensitive skins with sun exposure thanks to its soothing effect.

Donkey's milk soap: This is one of the best hidden secrets of Mexican brujas for glamour and beauty magic. Historical records show that donkey milk was often used as a treatment to revitalize the skin. Cleopatra, Queen of Egypt, was regarded as a great beauty, and it is said that she regularly took baths in donkey's milk. It is believed that Pauline Bonaparte, Napoleon's sister, brought the beauty secret of donkey milk to Mexico, since she also used it to care for her skin. Today, donkey's milk is a common beauty practice among brujas de rancho.

Honeybee soap: This soap is used to attract love and harmony. Use it to sweeten people's feelings toward you and your own attitude toward life. Rich in beeswax and alpha hydroxy acids, honeybee soap returns a smooth appearance to the skin.

Jabón-Zote soap: A favorite of Mexicans, this classic soap has a lot of history, magic, and folklore. With its unmistakable white color and aroma of citronella, it has accompanied Mexican daily life for generations. In addition to being very useful in washing and removing stains from clothes, this peculiar bar soap has shown multiple benefits and uses, such as the treatment of acne, as an insect repellant, an eliminator of common plant pests, and many more.

Maja soap: This is a soap to seduce the world. Thanks to its formula of essential oils extracted directly from the most beautiful flowers, it provides a sensual aura that favors friendship and romantic love. Maja soap can be used to attract love and harmonize environments.

Rosa Venus soap: It is not a surprise to find Rosa Venus soap in every motel in Mexico. Venus is known as the planet of love, and this soap is associated with love, passion, beauty, grace, charm, pleasure, sensuality, erotism, romance, and sex. For best results, it is recommended for use before and after love making.

Sulfur soap: Sulfur is a mineral used in spells to drive away negative people or energies. Sulfur comes from the Latin *sulphur*, which means "to burn." Sulfur soap is used to ward off negative or malicious forces attracted to your environment by sorcery or witchcraft, destroying them and forming a protective barrier around your body. This soap is also an effective anti-acne care. However, this soap tends to leave your skin very dry after its use, and is not recommended for daily use. Always use a humectant body cream after you use it.

Soap Spell to Diminish an Enemy

Use this spell to lessen the authority, dignity, and reputation of an enemy and make them meek. You will need:

> Jabón-Zote soap
> A mason jar with lid
> Water
> Paprika
> A toothpick
> Your own spit

On a Saturday night, take your Jabón-Zote soap and carve it into a figure of your intended target. Once you are happy with your figure, carve your enemy's name and date of birth into your soap. Place it on a plate and sprinkle some paprika on it, then repeat the following prayer:

> *In the name of the Father, the Son, and the Holy Spirit. Oh, powerful zote, help me to dilute, diminish, and banish my enemy, so (enemy's name) can't do any wrong against me. Get rid of all the evil that is found around me, dilute my opponent and prevent (enemy's pronouns) from doing any harm unto me. Undo my enemy from wishing me to fail. Amen.*

Spit on the soap three times and place the soap in the mason jar. Add water and close the jar. Place the mason jar somewhere dark where no one will see it. Allow the soap figure to dissolve in the water. When your figural representation has dissolved completely, throw the water out in a cemetery, and watch your enemy fall.

Rancho Remedies for Spiritual Diseases

When brujos de rancho refer to ourselves as Catholic, we do so in our own way, distinct from the institution, away from dogmas, "values," and norms. Some forms of adapted beliefs and practices are very different from the ones the Catholic hierarchy proposes, such as brujeria, hechicería, divination, necromancy, and taking justice into one's own hands. Among rancho folk beliefs, "God's law" means something entirely different from the church's law. Our beliefs and traditions are rooted in agriculture and ancestral beliefs, two concepts that are deeply intwined with each other. Like the saying goes, whatever man sows, he will also reap.

Even in pre-Hispanic times, among indigenous groups from different areas, such as the Nahuas, diseases were considered a punishment from the Gods, aimed at those who committed certain offenses. For example, Tlaloc and his assistants, the tlaloques, produced diseases related to water, cold, and humidity; Macuilxochitl sent ailments of a sexual nature; Nanahuatzin produced various ailments in the eyes.

Spiritual diseases are those ailments that make us feel incapable and trapped. They destroy our body and our spirit. People on the rancho are always working to better themselves and their community. They understand that spiritual diseases affect not only our bodies, but also everyone else around us. In this section, we discuss some common spiritual ailments and how to fight them the rancho way.

Susto

Susto in Spanish literally means "fright" or "scare." This phenomenon is also known as *cibih* in the Zapotec language. In Mexico, susto is understood as something that most affects children, although it can impact anyone of any age. Susto is caused by a severe fright. Symptoms may appear any time from hours to days after the fright is initially experienced, and it's believed that, in extreme cases, susto may even cause death. In traditional Mexican pre-Hispanic medicine, it is also considered "the loss of the soul." Susto has no "official" list of symptoms, as they vary from person to person and can include changes in appetite and sleeping patterns, pallor, and unusual bouts of daydreaming. The affected person always seems distracted or depressed. Susto may seem closely related to major depressive disorder or post-traumatic stress disorder. The DSM-5 includes susto in its categorization of cultural concepts of distress.

According to the traditional medicine of Mexico, it is advised that patients suffering from susto eat bolillo. A bolillo is a small loaf of plain white bread, crusty on the outside with a soft interior. The fright manifests more severely in the stomach, increasing gastric juices, so it is not advisable to have an empty stomach when you are suffering from susto; bolillo helps to settle the stomach. The indigenous Otomi people advise using stale bolillo. The harder the bolillo the better because the bolillos absorb the susto like sponges.

Susto Remedy with Two Bolillos
This is a remedy to clean susto from a person. In the rancho tradition, the treatment of susto must take place without the patient's knowledge. This remedy should be performed while the patient is sleeping.

It must be said that no single treatment cures all forms of susto, just as no one event causes everyone to suffer from susto, but this is by far the best method I know among the ranchos in Mexico.

You will need:

Two bolillos
Holy oil or olive oil
A stove or fire pit

Lay the two bolillos in a cross shape for three minutes, then anoint a cross on each of them with the oil. Anoint a cross on the patient's fontanelle as well. With each cross you anoint, say: *In the name of the Father, the Son, and the Holy Ghost.*

Afterwards, pass one of the bolillos in the form of a cross over the patient's sleeping body. (People suffering from susto tend to shake and a move a lot, even in their sleep.) Pray a credo three times while you do so. Take the bolillo and burn it until it gets black and ashy and throw away the charred remains in a sealed bag in the trash.

The next morning, the patient must eat the other bolillo.

Remedy for Envy

Envy is a form of sadness, regret, or pain caused by the qualities, possessions, or luck of others, the desire to possess something that you are lacking and that another possesses. The hostility and aggressive feeling experienced by the envious for those who enjoy something is presented as intolerance for the success of others, since the achievements of the envied often are not acknowledged or admitted. Both suffering and courage can upset the one who envies, giving rise to a desire to harm the one who is envied. The one who feels envy doesn't really want to win, after all—they want the one who is envied to lose.

To protect yourself from the envy of others, carry a small circular mirror in your purse or wallet. Consecrate this mirror by praying the following prayer:

> *My lord, kneeling before you, I pray that through the interces-*
> *sion of the Holy Spirit, my loved ones who loved me so much in life,*
> *my ancestors who I didn't get to meet, and all the saints and folk*
> *spirits that I'm devoted to, form around me a powerful circle pro-*
> *tector against envy, that the envious person reflects in this mirror,*
> *and that their envies only reflect their path, and not mine. Amen.*

Remedy for Gluttony

Gluttony is characterized by an excessive and ongoing eating of food or drink, which can cause *empacho*, a folk illness wherein food gets stuck to the walls of the stomach or intestines, causing an obstruction. It is thought to be caused by dietary indiscretions, such as eating too much food or spoiled food, inappropriate combinations of food, or eating at the wrong time. Most empachos can be prevented with this remedy. Gluttony is often nothing more than the result of an emotional void that the affected person is attempting to fill by giving into gluttony instead of facing the void.

A remedy for this condition is to practice moderation and fill the void with more emotionally fulfilling activities, such as going for a walk, visiting your family, and doing social service. If this doesn't help, carry around your neck a wooden crucifix. It is important that this crucifix be made out of wood. Wood is a material that allows a spiritual connection between people and the Divine; it is a natural symbol, considered to be an incredibly spiritually valuable material all around the world. Wood is often used to symbolize man, especially in his mortality, and the connection with the divine. It is no wonder that wood was the chosen material by the Lord himself. I have found that this remedy works better to fill the emotional void than behavior like compulsively shopping, smoking, drinking, or betting.

CHAPTER SEVEN

LIMPIAS AND HOME CLEANSINGS

"No andes descalzo que te vas a enfermar"
which translates to "Don't walk around barefoot or you will get sick."

—popular Mexican mom saying

A limpia is a ritual process that impacts favorably on our spiritual matter. One peculiarity of the limpias is their power of protection and their ability to remove unwanted energies from the environment. In some cases, the limpias can serve as shield-making sessions; these shields are energetic defenses against evil intentions, evil spirits, ill intent, and witchcraft against us.

The pre-Hispanic belief was that everything in the world had a spirit, and so hundreds of those spirits were asked for their intervention. The rituals that we as Mexicans have where we rely on the spirit world to clean, purify, and protect ourselves as well as remember our origins so that we shape our destiny positively, are products of the syncretism of so many different cultural inheritances and so they are among the most important.

In Mexico, cleanliness goes hand in hand with devotion and tradition. Just as people should be cleansed, so should objects, property, money, and jewelry be cleansed. The cleansing of material things is extremely necessary and important because sometimes the excess of envy, greed, jealousy, and the Evil Eye that these objects absorb can affect the owner of them.

There are many ways to prevent and remove evil and psychic disturbances. Sometimes we complicate our lives by finding needlessly complex remedies, when the ranch witches had extremely effective and simple methods to combat these threats. These practices can be done at home and in our businesses, workplaces, or offices. It is often enough to modify the prayers a little so they fit our needs. Even through the daily cleaning of these places, we can carry out a spiritual and energetic cleansing. In order to be properly spiritually cleansed, they must be swept and mopped properly.

Before doing a limpia in the house, on an object, on ourselves or someone else, the first step is that the person, object, or space has to be physically clean. Dirt, clutter, and mess make the energy heavy and static, so it is necessary to clean thoroughly. When my grandma did limpias for other people's businesses or houses, she never gave the service unless the place was physically clean.

You must choose a day when you feel good, physically and mentally. Your own energy is important in the process of cleansing a house. Open the windows and ventilate the whole house well. Cleaning should be done during the day and with the windows open. If there are curtains or blinds, they must be open to let in the light. Maintain a happy and optimistic attitude while you clean, this is highly important!

You can even use background music to improve your mood. (That's a very Mexican tradition right there!) If you do put on music, try to keep in mind that you should listen to lyrics that have to do with your purpose. If you are doing a limpia, please do not listen to "Paquita la del Barrio or anything resentful or about grudges." I know we can get the strength to clean when we are pissed, but this is contraindicated for a limpia.

Always start in the room farthest from the entrance of the house. Open the taps for a few minutes, let the water run, clean the toilets. Place everything in its rightful place, and sweep and remove as much dust as you can from the house. Move the furniture around, and donate or give away everything that you do not need or use anymore. The place must be neat physically before you perform a spiritual limpia.

When this type of cleansing is put in place, you should always use protection, as you would in spiritual cleansing for people in removal workings. The tetragrammaton (discussed on page 88) is an excellent protection for these purposes.

Sweeping: Saint Martin de Porres's Magic Broom

Since pre-Hispanic times, the purpose of sweeping was to purify and renew. It was done with the intention of starting a new cycle, with reverence to the gods, and to clean our path. Sweeping in Brujeria de Rancho is both essential and easy to do. In Mexican culture, sweeping becomes magic: it cleanses pride, sorrows, pain, anguish, and evil.

This is one of my grandma's favorites, Saint Martin de Porres's broom. Martin de Porres (November 9, 1579-November 3˙ 1639) was born in Lima, Peru, to Juan de Porres, the governor of Panama, and Ana Velasquez, a freed slave of African and Indigenous Panamanian descent. Martin entered the Third Order of the Dominicans when he was fifteen. He was devoutly religious and helped establish an orphanage and hospital. He was canonized as a saint in 1962. The broom is one of the most representative symbols not only of Saint Martin de Porres, who was nicknamed Brother Broom in his life, but also the action of sweeping and cleaning. The broom was the magic wand of San Martin de Porres. Once, someone asked San Martin de Porres: "And why, being so holy and miraculous, doing so many wonders, are you the one who sweeps the convent?" He replied: "By sweeping the convent, I direct the convent."

Brooms are emblems as well for brujos de rancho. Compartments with combinations of herbs, oils, prayers, holy images, words, and a variety of other things are known to have been part of spells and rituals for generations, hidden in the shaft of some rancho brooms.

The first thing we have to understand is a basic concept: what is a magic broom? A magic broom literally cleans not only physical dirt, but also etheric dirt. Magic brooms are used at the beginning of a ritual or a hechizo to cleanse the energies in the area where you are going to work. They are also used in your home or business as either prevention or necessary spiritual cleaning.

To create your magic broom, you will need:

A new broom, preferably with a wooden handle
Olive oil
Saint Martin de Porres prayer candle or a white or purple candle
Holy Water
A black permanent marker.

On a Tuesday, grab your new broom and draw a little mouse on the handle. After you've completed your drawing, sprinkle a little Holy Water on the brush of the broom. The bristles in traditional rancho brooms were made from corn or horsehair, but in modern brooms, they're commonly made from plastic. Don't worry about it, just follow the mechanics.

Next, rub a little olive oil on the shaft of your broom. Light your Saint Martin de Porres prayer candle and leave the broom in velacion, close to the candlelight. Say the following prayer three times:

> *Martin de Porres, humble follower of the Gospel of Jesus, we lift before you our hearts full of trust and devotion. You who with love gave yourself to the poor and helpless, today I come to you with my needs and requests. Dispense on us and on our families all blessings, remove from this place with your blessed broom what does not serve us, all envy, all evil intent, and all disease. O blessed Saint Martin de Porres, humble servant of the Lord, you filled the hearts of the needy, of the most disadvantaged, and you were the consolation of souls and bodies, you took great care of the sick, and you worked thousands of wonders and great miracles to favor those who came to you asking for help, I beg you to be our intercessor and, with your holy broom, sweep away all evil from this place. Amen.*

Leave the broom close to the candle until the candle is consumed. Please be aware of fire safety: do not put your broom so close to the candle that it is in danger of catching on fire. Afterwards, your magical broom is ready to be used.

Floor Washes

Floor washes are the traditional preferred method for spiritually cleansing a house. They are used to remove negativity, banish entities and bad spirits, remove brujeria, wash away bad luck, and bring increased customers and/or good luck in the home.

My grandmother used to say that most of the evil spell work done against people comes from the very individuals they've allowed into their homes. It can be a family member or someone who claims to be a friend. She also used to tell me that the easiest way to put an evil spell work into someone's home is with your shoes, sprinkling the spell work in question on the soles of your shoes before entering the other person's home. Yes, it's great to burn incense to cleanse the air in your home, but what about what's on the floor? This is especially a problem for those of us in cultures where we go barefoot at home.

Cleansing your home with these very traditional recipes is one of the most effective ways to get rid of hexes and clear the house. Usually powders, maledictions, and *salaciónes* come to our house traveling on our feet. You can also get rid of any dark spirits or attachments with these traditional formulas. These formulas are designed to be affordable and practical for the busy person who is already working two or three shifts to make a living, and who does not have enough time to make elaborate floor washes. These will not take a lot of your time or much money, but they will improve your life in a lot of ways!

Pine-Sol Floor Wash

For this floor wash, all you need is Pine-Sol Disinfectant Liquid All-Purpose Cleaner, better known in the Mexican world as PINOL, an ocote cross, and a bucket full of water. If you live somewhere where you cannot get Pine-Sol brand cleaner, another brand will do, but you must make sure it is made with real pine fragrance and not synthetic. Pour three caps of pine cleaner into your water-filled bucket and place your ocote cross inside. In the morning, clean your house with the water while praying the following Prayer of the Beautiful Wood Cross prayer.

Prayer of the Beautiful Wood Cross

The cross where Jesus had his last moments of life is a pillar of faith. It is necessary to understand the power of the cross: there is no sin, no plot, no evil spirit, no harm that cannot be cleansed, since the cross means life.

> *Oh! Ocote cross! Beautiful wooden pine cross where Jesus died to give us eternal light and free us from the enemy, before you I humble myself and reverently implore my Lord Jesus Christ that because of the sufferings that he received on you in his Most Holy Passion grant us the spiritual cleansing of this place and destroy all threats, witchcraft, all evil intents from this house and from all of who live in it. Amen.*

Fabuloso Lavender

There is nothing more Mexican and more traditional than lavender Fabuloso. The word lavender comes from the Latin *lavare*, meaning "to wash." For this wash, you are going to need an already blessed Palm Sunday Cross and three caps of purple Fabuloso, along with a bucket and water. Fill the bucket with water, add your three caps of Fabuloso, and place the cross inside it. Let it rest for the whole night and in the morning clean the house with it while saying the following prayer:

In the name of Jesus Christ, I raise this prayer to protect and clean my home. Merciful Lord, I ask you that if anyone wants to hurt my household or bring some evil or calamity here, to remove this person with no mercy. May their footsteps return to their destiny and not set foot in my house. Amen.

Tips for Magical Home Cleaning

Always pour the dirty water down the drain and do not use it to sweep the street! Wash your mop clean, never leave it dirty. Wear plastic gloves to avoid getting anything negative on your hands and wash the gloves in your cleansing solution before removing them if you plan to use them again.

If you live in a city in the USA or another part of the world where most homes are carpeted—not exactly rancho style—you basically have two options when it comes to floor washes. You can prepare these same solutions and use a spray bottle to mist your carpets, repeat the prayers, and then vacuum. (Check your vacuum's instructions to make sure it can handle damp carpets.) Alternatively, and this is my favorite, buy a powdered carpet cleaner and mix a little ground pine or lavender into it. (Make sure it isn't dyed and won't stain your carpet.) Sprinkle this mixture on your carpet, repeat the prayers, and vacuum the area. The same safety instructions apply to your vacuum: keep it clean, use gloves when you are cleaning, and remove the vacuum bag or the bin contents from your house.

Limpia with Candles

Fire is a powerful and accessible element. The simple act of lighting a candle can cause a significant change in the energy of a place. A flame lit with a specific purpose and following the guidelines of a well-defined ritual positively alters the dynamics in your home. Candles have a variety of religious meanings, especially for Catholics. A candle symbolizes that there is light even in the darkness. Candles detoxify the atmosphere of energetic darkness, returning harmony and warmth to the environment.

Limpia with Seven Archangel Prayer Candle

Archangels are the highest rank of angels. Some sources disagree about how many of them exist, but the most commonly referenced number in Mexico is seven. These angels keep an eye on humans and are associated with different aspects of existence. While all of them are wise, powerful guides and spiritual healers, they each have specific traits that apply to different situations. One of my favorite limpia with candles is the seven archangel prayer candle.

This limpia is performed for seven days, as every angel has a day and a color that represents them. If you can't find a seven archangel prayer candle, buy a seven-color candle and with a sharpie write the name of each angel in their color, or print an image of the seven archangels and glue it to the glass. Please get creative, never stop your magic because you can't find something.

Beginning on a Monday, light the candle and pray the following prayer every day for seven days. Each day, let the candle burn until one color has been consumed, and start with the next color the next day.

Seven Archangel Limpia Prayer

> *I (your name) call on the names of the seven archangels: Archangel Michael, Archangel Raphael, Archangel Gabriel, Archangel Uriel, Archangel Barkiel, Archangel Tzadkiel, Archangel Jophiel! I command you to banish all enemies from my presence, property, and family. Destroy every evil influence around me— no matter its form—in the underworld, in the air, in the ground, and in the water. Deliver me from those entities that fly and from those that crawl, and from all beings that would ever want to do me harm. Protect me, seven archangels. Mighty God, make your warrior angels strip those evil witches from all their psychic and occult powers. Strip them of their psychic visions, their abilities, and any*

other skills that allow them to attack me or have an advantage over me, so they do not harm me by day, so they do not harm me by night. Empower me to identify them. Guard me in my dreams and in my sleep. Remove all obstacles from before me and give success to the work of my hands. By the power of the Lord God Almighty. Amen.

Once the candle has been totally consumed, use the glass sleeve as a vase to offer flowers to the seven archangels.

Sahumerios

Sahumar (sow-mahr) means to perfume, to flood a space with smoke. This practice consists of burning herbs, resins, woods, powders, and flowers on a lit charcoal or a bundle. (Always use a bowl suitable for high temperatures.) The smoke that comes out of this junction is distributed throughout the space that needs to be purified. It is a very effective method to clean and protect from evil.

The main use of a *sahumerio* is to cleanse a place with the use of smoke produced by certain essences, resins, and herbs. This produces a clean environment free of negative entities and frequencies, and generates a feeling of peace while attracting wellness. Sahumar mobilizes energy, so it doesn't get stagnant. Burning resins and herbs also has a symbolic meaning that helps elevate our prayers and communications with spirits for the purpose of a ritual or magic working.

Sahumerio Against Envy

For this cleansing, you will need:

Wormwood
Blessed palm
Frankincense
Charcoal
A heat safe bowl

Once the charcoal is ready, add the wormwood, blessed palm, and frank-incense. As the smoke begins to rise, repeat the following blessing:

> *Any evil seed of envy cohabiting with my blessing, I uproot you by smoke and fire, every trick of the envious against me, my family, my job, or my property, will be exposed now in the name of Jesus. Amen.*

Resguardos: Home Protections

The Magic Doormat

My grandmother used to say that the best brujeria is the one that nobody notices. There are numerous ways to work protection magic for our home, but this has always been one of my favorites: the magic doormat. The pro-cess of passing your feet over a doormat is automatic, an act that not only has to do with hygiene but also has had magical connotations since ancient times. In many native tribes in Mexico, the mat was consecrated, a piece of cloth placed before the entrance to a sacred space.

To consecrate your own magical doormat, you will need:

A new doormat
A Saint Benedict key medal or medal (this version of the
miraculous Saint Benedict medal is specifically for
the home and meant to hang on doorknobs)
Red ribbon
Two white candles
Rosemary
Cinnamon
Oregano

The Saint Benedict medal is one of the most popular among Catholics. Saint Benedict is known for the power he holds over the devil, using the Holy Cross as his instrument to make the devil flee. Spiritual benefits associated with the pious use of this medal include warding off evil and temptation, obtaining the conversion of sinners, assistance for women during childbirth, strength in the preservation of purity, granting the grace of a happy death, protection during storms, and cures for diseases.

First, place your doormat in between the two candles. Lay the Saint Benedict medal on top of the mat. Light the right candle and say:

> By the power of God and the hand of Saint Benedict, the protection for this home and to those who enter it be manifested.

Light the left candle and say: With this medal/key, all negativity, bad vibration, or ill intent of anyone who enters this house is left outside this door.

Leave both candles lit until they have been fully consumed. Sprinkle the cinnamon, rosemary, and oregano on the mat and let it rest for seven hours, then shake it off. Pray the *Gloria Patri* five times:

> Glory be to the Father, and to the Son, and to the Holy Spirit,
> as it was in the beginning, is now, and ever shall be, world without
> end. Amen.

The mat is now ready to be placed at your threshold. The medal should hang inside your home either on top of your door or on the doorknob to fulfill its purpose.

Saint George's Sword Door Protection

For this home protection, you will need:

A Dracaena trifasciata (Saint George's sword) plant
Holy Water
A clay pot
Potting soil
A Saint George medal
Red ribbon

Place your Saint George's sword plant in the clay plot and cover it carefully with soil before watering it with the Holy Water. String the Saint George medal on the red ribbon and tie it gently onto one of the plant's leaves. Repeat the following protection prayer:

This household is dressed and armed with Saint George's sword so that our enemies having feet will not reach any of us; having hands will not trap us; having eyes will not see us, neither with thought can they cause us any harm. Firearms will not reach this place; knives and swords will break without passing this door. Jesus Christ protects and defends this place with the power of His Holy and Divine Grace. The Virgin of Nazareth covers this household with her sacred and divine mantle. And God, with His Divine Mercy and great power, is our defender against the evils and persecutions. Glorious Saint George, in the name of God, extend to us your shield and your powerful sword, defend us with your strength and your greatness; and may our enemies underneath your feet become humble and submissive to you. So be it in the Power of God, of Jesus Christ, and of the Divine Holy Spirit. Amen.

Cédula de San Ignacio de Loyola

Saint Ignatius of Loyola takes care of his devotees from the snares of the devil, bad influences, bad company, and people with bad intentions. He is a saint who spiritually battled with the Evil One and defeated him. Images and *cedulas* (prayer cards that contain a powerful exorcism) of San Ignacio de Loyola are placed on the back of doors in homes of the pious so that the devil cannot enter their rooms.

Saint Ignatius possessed an extraordinary ability to cry, especially while he was praying. His tears were always accompanied by a great sweetness. Because of the abundant flow of his tears, he could no longer pray the breviary; the tears even became so copious that they were collected in a pot. In remembrance of this gift, there is even today the custom of blessing water in altars dedicated to the veneration of him. Water of San Ignacio is blessed on July 31 of each year and is used for the protection of both home and business, to ward off negativity, and to keep the devil from doing his thing. You can use it in floor washes or home cleaning sprays. It's important to remember that both the certificate and the water work only if one has faith.

San Peter's Door Enchantment

You will need:

Holy Water
An image or prayer card of Saint Peter
Tape
Spray bottle
One camphor tablet
Red ribbon
A small key

Pour the Holy Water into the spray bottle, then add the camphor tablet and close the container. Tape the Saint Peter image or prayer card to the front of the spray bottle. String the key on the ribbon and knot the ribbon three times around the top of the bottle, once each for the Father, the Son, and the Holy Ghost.

Spray the inside and outside of your door while visualizing how the energy sent by the power of your word along with the Holy Water activates your protective door. While you spray, repeat the following prayer:

> *In the name of Saint Peter, the saint who is spiritually hold-*
> *ing the keys at the entrance of my place, I enchant this door with*
> *God's light so love and prosperity will grow every time this door*
> *opens. Hate and the Evil Eye will perish every time this door gets*
> *closed. I seal and protect with the power of the blood of Jesus Christ,*
> *this house with all that it is, with all that it has. I seal and protect*
> *the front door in such a way that all who enter and exit feel deeply*

protected. When someone calls on this door, this spell will increase its power by seven times. I seal and protect with the most precious Blood of Jesus Christ the Lord, all the walls, ceiling, corners, each one of the columns, and through them, I seal and protect the four cardinal points of this house. I seal and protect with the power of the Blood of Jesus Christ the Lord all the foundations from which this house was built. Peace, love, and joy grow in this place behind this door, with Saint Peter and God's blessing. Amen.

After that, tape the Saint Peter image on your door and leave it there. Do this hechizo preferably on the seventh day of the month. I usually do this on July 7 and it works amazingy.

CHAPTER EIGHT

LA IGLESIA Y EL CAMPOSANTO

I don't know what it is about the flowers, Llorona
The flowers of El Campo Santo
I don't know what it is about the flowers, Llorona
The flowers of El Campo Santo.

La Llorona—Mexican Folktale and song

There are certain things within Brujeria de Rancho that are not openly touched on social networks, not even among brujas. It is as if it were a deal that we have agreed between those of us who practice not to make certain information available. This magical secrecy did not happen voluntarily but was forced by political and sociocultural issues. But it is in our judgment when and for what reason we reveal those aces up our sleeve—aces that should be removed only in extreme situations.

The metaphor "the brighter the light, the darker the shadow" can be understood as being about balance. The more "good" that comes into existence, the more "evil" must come into existence as well. Brujeria de Rancho understands there is not one without the other and that the denial of evil is exactly what it fuels and causes it to become out of control.

The bruja de rancho is comfortable with her duality. There is no day without night. If only day existed, we would have some benefits, but they would be outweighed by problems for ecosystem. The same lack of balance would apply if only night existed as well. Therefore, believing that it would be better if only day existed is impossible, as is thinking that it would be better if only night existed. You may like one more than the other, but both exist and are essential for balance. The two parts are essential.

If we can look at things from a broader perspective, we can see that the sun and the moon exist at the same moment, although only one might be visible in the sky at any given moment. My grandma used to say that la bruja belongs to two places: la iglesia (the church) and el camposanto (the cemetery). I know some of you must be thinking, "But what could a bruja be doing in a church?"

La Iglesia: The Church

Those who have been exposed truly and directly in Brujeria de Rancho and its culture know well that this is something we do not talk about for several reasons. The first reason is because knowledge is power. Traditionally, this was the only power we had over the oppressive ways and norms, and we didn't intend to give it away. The second reason is for fear of excommunication. The information that I'm about to provide to you is a direct ticket to excommunication: these practices are infamous, sacrilegious, and dangerous. They are not to be taken lightly. Tools and rituals are a powerful source of magic, and the most important for a bruja are the ones that have to do with initiation, Baptism, Confirmation, Eucharist, marriage, and the Last Rites meant for preparing the soul of the dying person for death.

Sacramentals

Sacramentals are some of the least understood and most misrepresented elements of folk Catholic beliefs. Sacramentals are objects or actions blessed by a Catholic priest. Some examples of sacramentals are Holy Water, rosaries, crucifixes, medals and statues of saints, holy cards, and scapulars. The power of sacramentals, then, depends greatly on the devotion of both the priest who gives the blessing and the person who is receiving the sacramental.

Sympathetic Magic: Dolls, Fetiches, and Pictures

Among tourists in Mexico and other people who are foreign to our culture, the most frequently asked question about brujeria is, does it work? The answer is yes, if you are a bruja and you know what you're doing. Mexican brujas have the power to cause injury, harm, and disease without having to get close to someone; we dominate the dark arts and understand how sympathetic magic works.

Sympathetic magic is a form of magical ritual using objects or actions either resembling or symbolically associated with the event or person over which influence is sought. Nowhere was the cord between man and spirit more tightly bound than in the making of *amatl* (a Nahuatl word; *amate* in Spanish), the sacred paper of the pre-Hispanic peoples. Paper was sacred to both the Mayans and the Aztecs, along with other native cultures like the Otomi. It was the medium on which their history and the discoveries were chronicled, but it was also the material used to create *muñecos* (dolls) through a long-established technique of folding pieces of amate in half, then cutting them to the desired shapes. Even before the arrival of Spanish and African witchcraft, the use of dolls had centuries of history as a Mesoamerican tradition, using amate figurines for spells, cures, witchcraft, and other rituals.

Today, modern brujas can use pictures, dolls, and fetiches to represent a person. My grandmother and old-fashioned brujas usually preferred fetishes. "Fetish" derives from the Latin *factitius*, meaning "made by art." A fetish is an object believed to embody, be inhabited by, or attached to spirits. My grandmother was very rustic; she preferred to use older time-honored materials rather than modern ones, and so she would cut and sew the dolls. The goal is to create a doll that represents another person, so the more you personalize the doll, the better it will be. The thread, material, colors, and fillings used is totally up to you, but I advise to you to dress the doll with material that is similar to what the target tends to wear. Bonus points if you can get a piece of clothing from the person to bewitch and create your doll. If you are able to get a picture of your target, feel free to use one. Brujeria de Rancho relies on practicality.

Sacrament of Baptism

Once you have created a doll, tradition requires that the doll be administered the sacrament of baptism, even if the person we intend to bewitch may or may not have received it. In the past, the doll was exchanged by a wax figurine or a toad. It is highly important that you know the baptismal name of this person. A baptismal name, sometimes referred to as a Christian name, is a religious personal name that was historically given to a baby at their baptism. These days it is more often assigned by the parents at the child's birth. For the purpose of this ritual, we will refer to this name as the baptismal name as we hold a folk baptism for our doll. But why baptize the doll?

We receive a core identity upon baptism. Isaiah 43:1 says, "I have called you by name, you are mine." When you were born, you were given a name. According to folk Catholic faith, the name you were given at your baptism is your most important name, and it is with that name that you will give the fetish an identity.

For that, you are going to perform the folk version of a baptism. You will need:

The doll
The person's first name
Holy Water
Blessed paschal candle

Light the paschal candle and repeat the following prayer while you sprinkle the doll with a little bit of Holy Water: *I baptize you with the name of (say the name while focusing on that person) in the name of the Father, and of the Son, and of the Holy Spirit. Amen.*

The doll is now ready to use.

In case this person has had their confirmation sacrament or you know their patron or their protection saint

If this person has received the confirmation sacrament and you know their confirmation name or their patron saint, there are other things that can be done. When people decide on a confirmation name, the goal is to pick the name of a saint they admire, can relate to, or aspire to be like. This saint will be bonded to the person spiritually and in most cases is the one they turn to for guidance and protection, so you know which saint you are going to bind, tie up, and pretty much keep hostage locked in a matchbox until you are able to inflict the damage you intend on your target.

Requiem Mass

A Requiem or Requiem Mass, also known as the mass for the dead (in the Latin, respectively: *Missa pro defunctis* or *Missa defunctorum*), is a mass offered in the Catholic Church for the repose of the soul or souls of one or more deceased persons, using a particular form of the Roman Missal.

Traditionally, this work was conducted by first burying either the doll in the cemetery or in a jar filled with cemetery dirt and then going to a far-away church where the priest didn't know the target. Once there, you would ask the priest to perform a requiem mass using the target's name. Today, it is difficult to arrange a requiem mass for someone since it involves a lot of paperwork. However, in some churches, they will mention a name on a community requiem mass where you could easily write in that name to be added to the communal mass. In case that is not possible either, attend a requiem mass, and when the priest is mentioning the name of the deceased, you will say the name of your target discretely. A lot of brujos will sit in the front row so other people don't see them doing this. Usually the priest will not notice, as he is focused on performing the rituals.

To Cause Frigidity in Women

To introduce frigidity and uterine diseases to a woman so that she cannot crave anyone sexually, Mexican brujas use ball pins, sharp metal objects, and cemetery dirt. A doll is created that resembles the woman and the pins and cemetery dirt are inserted into the doll's vagina or into a cantarito (a pear-shaped jug) with the name of the target written on it. Cantaritos are an indispensable magical tool in Brujeria de Rancho. Cantaritos serve different purposes, from divination to one of the most infamous ones: to send a mal aire to someone.

In Brujeria de Rancho, everything has a correspondence to either a hot or cold polarity, including colors, shapes, and materials. A cantarito is a handmade pear-shaped jug made from clay pottery. Both the shape and the material of the cantarito are cold. The uterus is a hollow organ that is shaped like a pear, and interestingly has similar measurements and color to a cantarito, so a cantarito is useful in sympathetic magic involving the uterus. By keeping the uterus figuratively cold, the whole body is harmed. Among women who suffer from a cold uterus, many have chest problems, the most typical being fibrocystic breast, since the meridian that passes through the chest also contours the lower abdomen where the reproductive organs reside. That is, if the lower abdomen is "stuck" by the cold, it will also affect the breasts, along with a lack of lubrication, infertility, and frequent menstrual cramps.

To Send Mal Aire

When mal aires enter the human body, they cause terrible sickness. The Aztecs thought that certain people born on Ce-Ehecatl dates (the Nahuatl word for "One-wind" or "One-rain") gained supernatural abilities and that they had a special talent for malevolent magic. (This calendar differs greatly from the one in current use, and so the dates do not map exactly onto our calendar. They shift and rotate every year.) These individuals could change themselves into animals, or make people waste away and die or go mad. Ehecatl is an Aztec god of the air and winds, especially those that brought rain. Since the wind blows in all directions, Ehecatl is associated with all the cardinal directions and crossroads. There were several temples dedicated to Ehecatl, each of which had a unique form. They were pyramids, just like other Aztec temples, but instead of having quadrilateral platforms, they had circular platforms instead. The result was a cylinder-shaped structure. It's said that this form was intended to represent the deity as a fearsome aspect of the wind, such as a whirlwind or a tornado.

Wind is related to the underworld and sorcery in many cultures. On the Christian side, there is a long metaphorical tradition that associates cold and humidity with inertness, death, loneliness, sadness, depression, bad weather, and darkness. With this ritual, the symptoms of mal aire will appear unexpectedly on your target without apparent reason—they will suddenly "feel sick," beginning with a shooting pain usually in the back or lungs, stiffness in the neck, pneumonia, weakness, shivering, and severe episodes of depression. Mal aire can only be understood and healed based on the cosmogony and the beliefs of the particular ethnic or indigenous group in which it occurs. The cure for mal aire—or even exactly what mal aire is—varies in different parts of Mexico.

To send a mal aire, you will need:

A cantarito
A picture or doll to represent the target
Mecate or natural jute cord
Holy Water
A cleaning rag

The procedure is very simple. On a Saturday night, clean the inside of your cantarito with a rag and clean water. This ensures that the cantarito is free of any particle of dust and will introduce some humidity and moisture, which is the ideal state for this working. Introduce into your cantarito the picture or doll representing your target.

Once the picture or doll is inside the cantarito, place your two hands over the cantarito's opening, leaving just a small triangle of space. Blow into that space with all your strength seven times, creating a strong wind vortex. Once you have finished, take the cord and tie thirteen turns around the opening of the cantarito, envisioning as you do so a cerclage to close the opening. Leave this cantarito in a dark place away from the target.

El Campo Santo: The Cemetery

Since I was a child, I have always been drawn to cemeteries, especially for their energy and their art. The cemeteries in my hometown are beautiful, with many mausoleums that have been designed by renowned architects since 1899.

The first time I dabbled in this side of Brujeria de Rancho, I was nine years old. I remember it very well; it was the Day of the Dead and I had let go of my grandmother's hand while she prayed the rosary. I was lost for at least two hours and that was how I met Don Beto, the cemetery caretaker. He found me wandering near the north wing, where the oldest graveyards were. He smiled at me and told me that my grandmother was going crazy looking for me everywhere.

"Where have you been?" he asked. "What were you doing, *mija*?"

I innocently answered him that I was telling the spirits, at least those who names I could read, that they were remembered because sometimes I think about them, that I hoped they were at peace, and that I did not want them to feel alone, because their families had already let the grass grow and did not come to clean and that as long as I could come, I could pray to them and dust off their tombstone.

Don Beto gave me a look that was somewhat Machiavellian, but at the same time understanding and comforting. The only thing he said out loud was to himself. "Yes, when they are born with it, they realize it fast."

It took me a few years more to understand what he was talking about. Don Beto never saw me again with the same eyes, but he was always happy when I returned to the cemetery. The last time I saw him was when my grandmother passed away back in 2019. He came to give us his condolences, hugged me and whispered to me, "They are happy that you are here, you know."

My father believed that he was senile, but Don Beto and I understood each other with few words, and with those Machiavellian looks I developed after. Don Beto was one of my best allies to my craft, my eyes, and my key to the cemetery.

La Tierra de Panteon: Cemetery Dirt

According to Catholic eschatology, it is there in the *Campo Santo*, the cemetery, where the bodies rest until the day of judgment and resurrection. To heal or to kill that is the dual energy on the ground of a graveyard. In ancient times, certain topical medicines were extracted from the earth of specific mausoleums, such as the tombs of saints or those who died early, children or adolescents. These medicines had great healing and regenerative qualities for those still alive.

It is also well known that there is extremely negative and degenerative energy in some parts of the cemetery, especially where the bodies of people with sudden deaths or murdered without having getting justice lie, where their relatives come to fertilize this soil with their tears and bitter laments for them. This is not something to take lightly. If it is not done correctly, this can have serious consequences for the practitioner. If the person you are trying to reach is out of your league, if they have proper protective measures already in place, or if you are not doing this kind of trabajos for the right reasons. Even though Brujeria de Rancho as a tradition does not believe in karma, we do believe in balance.

Collecting Cemetery Dirt

It is necessary to clarify that taking dirt or anything else from a cemetery is not something that can be done lightly or arbitrarily; to do otherwise can bring disastrous consequences. Mal aire is commonly thought to be one such consequence, but these beliefs can and do vary greatly from place to place in Mexico. Where I come from, bad air is believed to be particularly dangerous: when it enters the body, it can cause illness or ruin.

Different Mesoamerican cultures believe that bad air emanates from corpses. *Ihiyotl* (Nahuatl for breath, respiration, and sustenance, the animating force) resides in the liver and often gives off mal aire by escaping from the body after death in gaseous form—think of the smell of decomposing bodies. It could then float around the cemetery as ghosts or phantoms, and get into living bodies through the orifices, like the nose, mouth, belly button, and other parts that we usually have covered by clothing. Brujas and brujos in the rancho cover their mouth, nose, and their tonalli (head) with a *rebozo* (a Mexican shawl) when they visit the cemetery to prevent the entering of evil air. Today, I use a black hoodie that covers everything. (These protective coverings must be black.) I advise you to follow my example: the easiest way to cover all your orifices is to use a shawl or a black hoodie, while your belly button should be covered with a red cord and an *ombliguera* (a Mexican obsidian navel stone).

The cemetery is not a place where people usually take their children, due to the exposure to mal aire, attachments, and spiritual attacks. My grandma did not worry much about me every time she had to do "her thing" at the cemetery, because she knew I knew how to handle myself, but she never took my sister.

Entierros: Burials

A burial in terms of Mexican witchcraft is a ritual done with the purpose of causing harm or obtaining something from someone. The goal is to make them feel suffocated, as if they were being buried. The burials performed in my grandma's time utilized toads, frogs, and even uteruses (which mostly came from cows). Today we use dolls, figural candles, photographs, clothing, and other personal belongings of our target, or even drawings with the target's name and date of birth of our target.

Burials can be done in a cemetery or in a witch's house using clay pots or glass containers filled with cemetery dirt, alcohol, and camphor. Burials require conjure and invocations to disembodied spirits or dark forces in order to achieve our mission. They should be made carefully; before doing a burial, always take into consideration collateral damages.

Trabajos de Amor y Domination: Love and Domination Spell with Burial
You will need:

A picture of your target
A very fine needle
Red thread (or red marker)

A Ziploc bag
Clay pot
Dirt
Water

Grab the picture of your target with your right hand and pass it all over your body five times, giving special attention to your private parts. Mentally repeat the following:

> *(Name of this person), just like I pass and rub your photograph all over my body, the same way you are going to crave this body, and you will not have peace or rest for as long as you do not come to me with all your soul, your body, and your heart, to give me your life and live it for me and only for me.*

Having said these words, take the finest needle you can find, fine enough so as not to damage the photograph, and thread it with the red thread. Stitch over the photograph's eyes, starting at the bottom up over the eyelids until the eyes are completely covered by red thread. (If you cannot do this, use a red marker to cover up the eyes instead.) Once you have completed this, repeat the following statement:

> *(Name of the person,) by the power of Lucifer, the Prince of Belzebuth, I sew your eyes, so that you have no peace or rest in any part of the world without my company and you remain blind for others (woman or man) so you can only see me and you can only think about me. (Name of the person), here in this pot I have you imprisoned and tied up so you cannot see the sun, the moon or the stars. Until you love me, you will not be able to live without my love and my caresses. I will not take you out of here, and if I take you out and you do not behave, here in the same pot I will put you back.*

Proceed to place the picture in a Ziploc bag and completely seal it. Bury the bag in a clay pot with dirt and a little water. Every Friday, water it a little and repeat the same prayer until your target comes to you. Keep the pot in your house. You can add a fake succulent on top; they look very real and no one will know what you have inside of that pot. Once your intended is with you, take the picture out of the pot. Put it back if your intended misbehaves.

Plantain Spell to Take Revenge on a Man Who Cheated on You

Although grown most frequently in the tropical coastal areas of the country, plantains are found in markets all over Mexico, where they are called *plátano macho*. They look like bananas on growth hormones, ranging in color from bright green and unripe to nearly black and overripe. In Veracruz, because of its strong Afro-Caribbean culinary and brujeria roots, plantains are used to create delicious dough for empanadas and for delicious black-bean filled croquettes, along with a variety of fritters and desserts. They are also used for trabajos to punish cheating men.

Cuquita was a well-known bruja in Veracruz who women used to visit for these specific workings. She was really good friends with my grandma. One day, she was visiting el rancho, and one of my aunts was crying, heartbroken over a cheater to whom she used to be married. Cuquita then taught this trabajo to my grandmother.

This is an irreversible spiritual working that renders its target sexually impotent. You will need:

A plantain (if you can't find one due the season or your loca-
    tion, you can use a regular banana)
Pork lard (you can use vegetal lard if you cannot han-
    dle pork for religious or dietary reasons)
A knife
Three black ball pins
Black ribbon, preferably wired
Brown paper
Black ink pen
The cheater's underwear

Red pepper flakes (Yes, the ones you use for pizzas and pastas!
Most red pepper flakes are a mix of peppers, with cayenne
taking up the majority of the share. The makeup may
change depending on brand, but they work wonders.)

Visualize in your mind the man you want make impotent. Think hard about him not being capable of having sex with anyone. Take the plantain in your right hand and visualize how his member is not even able to shake.

Take the knife and make a slit in the middle of the plantain. On the brown paper, write down the name and date of birth of your target. Insert this paper into the slit you cut in the plantain, then put some chile flakes inside the plantain. Take some of the lard and rub a little on the plantain, then sprinkle more chile flakes to cover it.

Take the three ball pins and place two in the form of an inverted cross in the middle of the plantain and the last one in what would be the tip of the penis or urethra. The urethra runs along the penis and opens at the tip. In addition to urine, it carries seminal fluid during ejaculation.

Wrap the plantain carefully with the cheater's underwear and tie everything together with the black ribbon, making thirteen tight knots without damaging the plantain. Once you have it ready, you are going to bury it at the cemetery or in a pot on your house with cemetery dirt. Repeat the following prayer:

In the name of the thirteen powerful purgatory souls, (name of
the cheater), from this day on, your sexual life is over. Your member
is death, as dead as the people laying in the cemetery. You will never
again have pleasure with any woman or with any man. There will
be no more sexual pleasure in your life for you.

To Cause Paralysis or Thrombosis

For this working, you will need a photograph of your target. Divide symmetrically in two a picture of your target, starting from the head to the crotch. Bury half of the photograph in the cemetery and place the other half on your altar. When you do this, the target loses strength and sensitivity in the middle of the body. By dragging one leg, one of the arms becomes inactive, and it makes it difficult for your target to speak, as when someone suffers from cerebral ischemia or thrombosis.

To Cause Alcoholism and/or Drug Addiction

Introduce a doll or a photograph of the target to a bottle with tequila or rum. That person will fall prey to uncontrollable desires to drink or anxiety about alcohol, and he will act in a disoriented and strange way. Some brujas in Mexico place marijuana, peyote, and even other chemical psychotropics inside the bottle to make the person crave those drugs.

Chapter Nine

THE PACT

Encendiendo una veladora a San Miguelito y otra al diablito.
Lighting a candle for Saint Michael and another to the Devil.

—Mexican folk proverb

According to traditional Mexican beliefs about witchcraft, a pact can be established between an individual and Satan, or another demon or demons. The individual offers either their soul or some other precious or valuable item in exchange for powerful and diabolical favors. These favors vary according to the demon and the desires of the person concerned.

The agreement can be oral or written. If oral, it is done through invocations, spells, or rituals: once the bruja de rancho believes that the demon is present, she asks for whatever favor she desires and offers something in exchange. The written pact includes a contract signed with different inks, often mixed with blood, herbs, and various colors.

Practitioners of Brujeria de Rancho have their own unique ways to pact, and their own entities according to our own folklore. The pacts are usually oral, through conjures, invocations, or prayers done on Tuesdays and Fridays, usually at midnight in isolated places, like *cerros* (hills). By covering up all religious paraphernalia such as crucifixes or saint statues, our homes or even a church can be used as a location while we pact or call upon those entities. Always take into account that there is an exchange with such entities. This is not a one-way deal.

Prayers and Conjures

The Mexican Inquisition changed established conceptions and norms in Mexico in two very important ways. The first is the domestication and feminization of the occult and magic. The rituals and worship that occurred, which had previously taken place mostly in the mountains, forests, rivers, and caves, from the sixteenth century onward were forced to survive in houses, to be done privately with the utmost secrecy. Likewise, the men who dominated the occult, magic, and sorcery were slowly displaced and replaced by women, who occupied and conquered those places. Conjures, pacts, and prayers by brujas de rancho were part of the popular culture, and transmitted from one woman to another. These conjures and pacts are more than refrains or formulas: they are prayers that the brujas de rancho pronounced with special fervor and adorned with an offering bow.

The Devil in the Ranch

This would not be a Mexican Brujeria book if I did not mention El Diablo, the devil, or El Chamuco. El Chamuco is a name for the devil used by people on the northeastern ranches. The word "Chamuco" comes from the Spanish *chamuscar*, which means to burn. This evil being's purpose, according to folklore, is to destroy the human beings, to tempt and seduce them. There are many legends surrounding the devil, and many names too: Satanas, Luzbel, the Prince of Darkness, El Chamuco. Whatever you want to call him, he is feared by some and venerated by others.

There are different ways to work with the devil in Mexico, but this is the ranch way. It begins with the story of a church in a municipality of Nuevo León; Sabinas Hidalgo, to be exact, where my grandmother Diana was born. Since old times, there has been a macabre legend, one that grandparents would tell their grandchildren. Inside the first chapel that was built in Sabinas, very close to the river, was a shrine dedicated to Prince Saint Michael Archangel, the head of the heavenly court, the same one who subdued the devil and who appears in old prayer cards, almighty with his flaming sword in his right hand and the scales of justice in his left—but often weighing the unlucky souls of people on these scales, as well. El Chamuco burns in the flames of hell and begs for mercy at the feet of the powerful chief prince of heaven.

Before the power of Saint Michael Archangel, many devotees prostrated themselves to request his protection from danger, for good health, money, love, and good crops and protection of their cattle. But the story goes that there were many who were not favored by the heavenly prince. Among them were witches from nearby rancherias. Desperate, they began to pray to El Chamuco inside of the church instead after their pleas to Archangel Michael had fallen on deaf ears. They turned in their despair to Satanas, and put their trust in the Prince of Darkness, who was, after all, also represented at the little church.

Suddenly, people of "bad reputation"—such as sex workers, witches, gamblers, and thieves—began to assist in the church. The little priest of the church even wondered, surprised, if perhaps Archangel Michael with his divine power had performed the miracle of attracting them to the holy place. One day, by accident, the altar boy overheard one of the new "faithful" —a woman who had a reputation as a witch in her region—say the following: "*Oye Chamuquito*, you who are next to San Miguelito, make my love, the *doctorsito*, love me, and ask my hand in marriage, so his father forgives my father the rancho debt of our land. Come on, do me that little favor and I'll offer you this little gift in exchange."

The "little gift" was a big cigar that she took out of her purse. This was the first prayer that the altar boy was able to hear and out of curiosity, he pricked up his ears and heard that the prayers being offered were not for San Miguelito, but for El Chamuco. Word of El Chamuco's compliance spread quickly and even people with good customs went to request favors, not from San Miguelito, but from the Chamuco, who granted revenge, money, love, and all kinds of requests quickly and efficiently.

One day the altar boy told the father what he saw and what he heard. The priest was incredulous, but he realized he could verify it once inside the confessional, hidden and spying on the parishioners. He listened to the prayers of the people who, instead of praying to the Divine Archangel, begged instead El the Angel Expelled from Paradise for favors. The priest decided to remove the image of the devil from the altar, although many in the town missed it.

Many people wondered where the image of the compliant prince had been sent. Local legends suggest that it was locked up for a long time—others say it was burned. To this day, many churches in this area only have statues of Archangel Michael that do not include the Devil.

To Ask El Chamuco a Favor

Find a Saint Michael church with a depiction of the devil underneath his feet. If you cannot find a church that fits the bill, or you have a problem going into a church for whatever reason, you can buy a statue of Saint Michael Archangel with the devil beneath his feet to put on your altar. I recommend doing this before buying a Chamuco statue, since these statues can be difficult to obtain in the US.

Cover the archangel with white fabric. Make your petition orally and do not forget to make an offering. Appropriate offerings include cigarettes, tequila, sotol, tamales, or a good cut of meat, such as a cowboy steak or a ribeye (if you can afford it; this is usually offered by people who raise animals).

El Charro Negro: The Black Charro

El Charro Negro is a supernatural being in Mexican folklore. The current version links the Black Charro with a representation of both the devil and a sinister version of Saint Martin of Tours. Among Mazatecs, the Black Charro is known as the owner of the land and the mountains. He is described as a handsome, tall young man, warm and friendly, with a white complexion and a friendly smile, dressed in an elegant black charro suit with silver spurs. He rides on a horse. Some nights, he comes down to visit his animals and keep an eye on treasures buried during the Mexican Revolution. Those who wish to obtain money from this being must go in a state of indulgence (sexual abstinence) and arrive with water and offerings for his horse.

Northern brujas say that El Charro Negro is actually the spirit of Agapito Treviño, who was considered the Robin Hood of Monterrey. Agapito was the fruit of a forbidden love; his father was a rich landowner and his mother an Indigenous woman who was mistreated by Agapito's father. At the age of eighteen, Agapito dedicated himself to robbery on the roads. He shared large parts of his thefts with the poor, mostly women and children. He became greatly famous as a robber and was the terror of the landowners who traveled in carriages.

According to Mexican folklore, the Black Charro appears at night, through the streets of cities or on rural roads. Being mysterious, he sometimes accompanies walkers, but if the person agrees to get on the Black Charro's horse or receives the sack of gold coins from him, that person's soul will take the place of the Black Charro as the devil's personal collector and watchman of the place.

Prayer to the Black Charro

> *O Lord of the Crossroads, who owns every single path, send your servant the Black Charro, patron of brujas del rancho, to come and raise his voice on this precipice where I find myself, to provide me with his help in my needs, that with his mercy he grant me power, good luck, and fortune. I ask you this with great faith and respect that my request be granted. I pledge your aid so I achieve and conquer what I need to achieve and conquer, so that my paths are smooth and full of opportunities, love, and wealth, open with clear vision, so that I never lack what I want, or what I need. O Great Black Charro, get rid of my enemies, and protect my life and my steps from evil, but especially grant me your powerful patronage. Amen.*

This prayer is to be said at a crossroads. Sometimes you may see the Black Charro, and other times you may feel a cold and humid wind travel through your bones. Some only smell him. Everyone has a different experience. Once you sense his presence, leave the water, cocoa beans, and some turkey as offerings. For a better understanding of this ritual and belief, I recommend this song: *Mi Padrino El Diablo* by Edwin Luna and La Trakalosa de Monterrey.

Prayer to Justo Juez Negro: The Black Just Judge

The Just Judge is an invocation of Christ (the word "just" in Spanish means righteous—the quality of being morally and spiritually correct or justifiable). His faithful believers come to him for his gift of justice, to ask him to keep enemies and violence away from their lives. He can also be asked to truly do justice in cases where someone is accused of a crime they have not committed. The black Just Judge is not recognized by any Christian church as he is said, according to Mexican folklore, to represent Satan.

The purpose of this prayer is for a woman to obtain the love of a man, forcing the will of the man in question by calling upon Lucifer, but you can also work with the Justo Juez Negro to get your way in court cases.

> *My Black Just Judge, just as you tame and weaken the young man, I want you to tame (say the person's name), don't let him sit in a chair, rest in his bed, or to be with a woman, so that he doesn't have a quiet moment. Lucifer, Lucifer, just like you led the four thousand souls to hell, I want you to lead (person's name), for me. If he is sleeping, do not leave him alone, fill his bed with thistles and fill his pillow with stones, do not leave him alone. With one of your devil's tails that is the longest there is, I want you to tie me to (person's name); he does not have peace of mind until he is completely united to me. I will pay you for all this by praying to you three times at midnight during nine nights. I promise to be thankful to you for this favor and spread this devotion, faith, and prayer to the first unfortunate woman or man in need of it. Amen.*

To Fix a Court Case in Your Favor

If you find yourself caught in a legal snare and you need to be found innocent, or at the very least not punished, perform this ritual. Leave your court papers under a black or Justo Juez Negro candle from midnight until three AM as you recite the following prayer with lots of faith.

> *Righteous Black Judge, I come to you for protection. Listen to this prayer, help me since I am very afraid of the adversities and sorrows that I am going through. Today I ask you to help me and allow me to get out of this terrible situation that anguishes and torments me and doesn't let me sleep. Lord, clear my case. Get rid of any person who can point a finger at me. I trust you, because I know you understand my complicated situation. I entrust to you my difficult case. (Here, you must speak to the Black Judge and explain your individual circumstances and the difficult case you are facing. Be detailed so the Black Judge can help you!) I place it in your hands so that you can defend me, hide me, and keep me safe from punishment. Oh Divine Judge! You, the one who renews my hope, the one who gives color to my cloudy situation, may they find in my favor, may I escape from punishment, make them set me free. Lord, hear my plea, do not forsake me. Amen.*

After the hearing is complete and the judge has found in your favor, light a second black candle for the righteous Black Judge, for the next thirteen consecutive Fridays during the same hours you lit the first one.

Los Polvos: Powders

The tradition of magic powders is as old as the world. There are ancient books in all cultures that speak of this type of trick. Powders are very practical. My grandmother used to say that the best Brujeria is the one that nobody notices, and one of the best ones is the powders.

But how do these powders work? It's very simple: when you prepare them, you transfer magical properties that belong to specific ingredients and ritualistic magic. Not all powders have the same purpose and not all are harmful, but most of them are very infamous., For example, there are love powders that you can spread in the bedsheets of your target in order to exert your control. When it comes to powders that cause harm, they must be managed very carefully. They are usually spread via the soles of shoes belonging to someone who has access to the target's home or business. Usually those powders act fast, since many people at home walk barefoot, and in Mexican folklore we understand that most physical and spiritual diseases enter through our feet. That's the reason why limpias and floor washes are so important. (See the chapter on limpias for more information.)

To make powders, you will need:

A molcajete or a pestle
Kitchen herbs and pantry staples such as salt and sugar
Cemetery dirt
Candles of different colors, representing different saints, and of
    different shapes according to the desired purpose

To make your base powder: Most brujas in Mexico use Maizena Corn Starch Unflavored or Tres Estrellas rice flour. These substances will make up half of your mix. It is the base to which you will add your herbs, cemetery dirt, and other elements. (Example: if you need a ¼ cup of powder, you are going to use two tablespoons of corn starch and other two tablespoons of the rest of the ingredients. A ¼ cup of powder would be enough for three workings, so now you have an idea how little the amount of powder you need to screw someone.)

To prepare the powder: Check the correspondence tables in the back of this book so you can plan the best time to create your powder and the proper color candle to use according to the purpose of your powder.

Have your base handy and ready to be mixed with the other ingredients. It is not recommended that you make two different powders the same day due to the risk of cross contamination of ingredients or energies. Light the proper color candle that matches the purpose of your powder; the color of the candle has an impact on the power of the powder as this powder is ritualized.

Place your first herb in the molcajete and powder it as finely as possible, visualizing your desire and your purpose as you look at the candle. Feel the energy that is transferred from your hands to the mortar.

Repeat the same action with each of the herbs. Consistency is of the utmost importance so that no one notices your powders; grind everything as finely as possible, until your ingredients are pulverized. Once you have ground all your herbs, mix the ingredients and add the cornstarch or rice flour to the mixture. This is the most important step of the ritual: when mixing the herbs with the cornstarch, recite the appropriate prayer and let the candle burn.

Store your powders in very small amounts in kraft paper treat size bags or small flat glassine waxed paper snack bags. It is important to label them with symbols that you are able to remember to avoid getting them mixed up.

Separation Powder

To end a relationship with the power of three graves.

Day: Saturday

Candle: Black

Base: Corn starch

Ingredients: Black pepper, dirt from the graves of three different people, Cal (calcium hydroxide, quicklime, or slaked lime), and rose thorns.

Prayer: *Oh, spirits of the three graves, three times I invoke your souls to help me with the mighty strength of Cain and the other graveyard spirits so couple (here say their names) does not have a future together and that all their plans, projects, and love fall apart, that they cannot be in the same place and that the spirit of hatred torments them every time they are together. Amen.*

Retiro, Alejamiento: Retreatment Powder

To be used to remove a person from your or another person's life.

Day: Saturday

Candle: San Alejo (Saint Alex)

Base: Corn starch

Ingredients: Garlic, alum stone, and a dry natural flower robbed from a graveyard.

Prayer: *Blessed San Alejo, I invoke you to use your abundant power to help me to remove this person from my life/the life of (name of the person). Keep this person away from me or (person's name). I beg you to influence (target's name), causing a strong desire in (target's name) to just walk away. If you comply with me, I promise to spread your miracle and repay this way, (here you make your offering to San Alejo). Amen.*

Love and Lust Domination Powder

Day: Friday

Candle: Santa Marta candle or red candle

Base: Rice flour

Ingredients: dried rose petals, jasmine, patchouli leaf powder (if you cannot get patchouli, use cinnamon).

Conjure: *I invoke and conjure Martha, not the worthy or holy one. Martha, come and bring (target's pronouns) to my bed so that without me (target's pronouns) can neither be nor rest. Martha, I conjure you with Barabbas, with Satan, with Volcanás, and however many devils are in hell. Martha, my luck fell on you, you have to bring it to me. (Name of this person), "With two I see you, with five I tie you, I drink your blood, with the outcasts of your mother's womb, your mouth I cover up, (name of the person) come to me humbly like the sole of my shoes."*

CHAPTER TEN

LENT FOR MEXICAN WITCHES

"Jesus, remember me when you come into your kingdom."

—Saint Dismas (the good thief, from Luke 23:42)

I t is common for witches to feel isolated during lent, or to isolate themselves from the traditions and celebrations of our Christian or Catholic families, especially if we have experienced religious trauma—and this is totally justified. Brujeria de Rancho works within certain religious frameworks and ways, so if you dabble in Mexican magic for long enough and want to go further with this tradition, that framework is something you are going to have to face eventually. Most Western folk magic traditions are Abrahamic in one way or another, but brujas de rancho managed to separate the dogma and the institution from the belief hundreds of years ago. It can even be said that, from a certain point of view, we are very cynical and only concerned about our own magic interests, typically disregarding accepted or appropriate standards for the Catholic Church in order to achieve them.

Although Holy Week in Mexico is a Spanish heritage, dating from the time of the conquest, the religious celebration integrates pre-Hispanic cultural backgrounds and traits that make it a festivity of profound religious syncretism. There is no precise date for its celebration, since it is subject to the full moon phase, for which the dates vary from year to year. According to Catholic tradition, Holy Week is the last week of the period known as Lent, which begins on Ash Wednesday and ends on Good Friday. During this period, seven Fridays of Lent must be fulfilled, since each one of them is dedicated to a religious dedication or passage from the period of the passion of Jesus Christ.

It is not a surprise that Mexican witches have developed a lot of traditions since Holy Week is loaded with meaning associated with astronomical cycles, with the duality of good and evil, excesses, life, and death.

Fat Tuesday o Dia de Carnaval

Fat Tuesday is the day before Lent begins on Ash Wednesday. This day became known as Fat Tuesday because of the tradition of a pre-Lent feast of pork, red meat, sex, and alcohol—the things that you are supposed to be willing to give up during forty days of Lent. On this day, Mexican witches go to the carnival or have good time drinking, eating yummy foods, and having fun.

Ash Wednesday o Miercoles de Ceniza

Ash Wednesday is the first day in the season of Lent. During Lent, we remember the forty days that Jesus spent in the desert being tempted by the Devil. Ash Wednesday also symbolizes the Christian belief that humans were created from dust, and we will return to dust and ash when we die. On Ash Wednesday, it is traditional to go to mass and receive the ashes.

Choose what do give up for Lent with a tarot or an oracle. My grandma always used her Spanish card deck and I use my tarot deck to communicate with the spirit about what we need to give up, or what would be a good offering.

Palm Sunday o Domingo de Ramos

Palm Sunday is the day on which Christians commemorate the triumphal entry of Jesus of Nazareth into Jerusalem, acclaimed by the crowd, days before his passion, death, and resurrection. The blessing of palms or olive branches is customary, commemorating this episode, from which comes the name of the festival. Its date is variable like Holy Week, but it is always celebrated on the Sunday before Easter Sunday.

Palm crosses are a powerful brujeria ally. A lot of people in the northern region of Mexico place a blessed palm cross inside of a clay cazo with water and leave it during overnight. They then use that water in the morning for baths, to sweep the streets, mop their floors, and even for food and tea preparation. Other people in the southern region of Mexico burn these crosses and use the ashes to make black salt for brujeria, for floor washes, amulets, and to protect people from Evil Eye.

I encourage you to get at least three to five palm crosses for your magical use for the year. Placing blessed palms with a prayer card behind the front or principal door of your home helps to drive away material and spiritual enemies, attracts blessings and health to the members of the house. This has been one of the most famous folk Catholic traditions in Mexico for centuries, and it works wonders.

Place blessed palms with a red ribbon in a baby's crib to prevent the Evil Eye, bad air, and drive away evil spirits.

Holy Thursday

This day aims to remind us of the journey and sacrifice of Jesus, from the place of the Last Supper to Mount Calvary, where he was crucified. From the night of Holy Thursday until the morning of Good Friday, it is a Biblical and Catholic devotion to visit seven churches, a very Mexican and mystical tradition, to visit seven temples or churches. The rancho tradition is to steal Holy Water from these seven churches. If you can't do this, try to buy Holy Water from seven different temples, or take your own water to them and the priest can bless it for you.

The mixture of the seven waters is extremely powerful for spell work, baños (spiritual baths), and floor washes.

Protections and Guards for Passion's Days

It needs to be said that the majority of brujas de rancho *do not* work on the Holy Week. However, there are some who work malevolent magic because the devil is loose on these days, especially from Friday after 3 PM until Sunday. These days are widely used to curse, hex, and mortally wound adversaries and enemies, so our grandparents taught us to protect ourselves from evil and jealous witches.

The most common and powerful protection is to take three sips of Holy Water and pray three Creeds. It is preferable to do this between midnight to 4 AM on Friday. These are legacies from our grandparents, who mostly respect these days, and use them to get everything we need to work for the following year.

Good Friday

On Good Friday, the Passion of Christ is remembered and commemorated with the Stations of the Cross, which in Latin means the way of the cross, and the ceremony of the Adoration of the Cross or *Via Crucis*

On this day, crosses in churches and home altars are covered with purple cloths as a sign of the absence of Jesus. The images are uncovered on Easter Sunday as a symbol of the Resurrection of Jesus.

The image of the Virgin Mary is dressed in black as a sign of her mourning and deep sorrow for the death of Jesus. Some brujas and hechiceras also dress in black clothing to symbolize mourning.

Nail Cross for Protection

On this day, before 3 PM, make a nail cross amulet for protection. They laid Jesus on the cross, spread his arms, and in each of his hands they nailed a large and sharp nail. The third nail nailed his two feet together. The nails mean lack of freedom. It means that the Lord paid the price for us to be free from all bondage. The nails symbolize our liberation. The first nail means that we are free from everything by his name. Jesus took the curse on that nail for us. The second nail means that in Jesus Christ, the arguments were canceled. The arguments are a legal right that was given to the adversary or enemy. This nail annuls the act of decrees, arguments, or curses that are held against us. The third nail means victory over oppression. It was embedded in the ankles of both feet. It means we should not live under oppression or curses. Christ has already paid the price for us to walk freely; he took that nail in his feet on the cross to cancel it.

This cross is very easy to make. You will need three nails, wire, and a little bit of imagination. This is something that is completely customizable; you can personalize your cross to your tastes.

Place a nail with the head up. Make a cross with the two remaining nails; make sure the nails are facing horizontal with the head of the nails out on both sides. Wrap the wire across them three times, making sure they're secure. When this is done, pray three Creeds.

At 3 PM on Good Friday, the crucifixion is remembered by praying the Apostles' Creed three times, as well as a rosary for Maria, Christ's mother, to meditate on her suffering. Give thanks to her for giving birth to the Savior.

I usually make my nail crosses on this day and they work wonders. You can place them on your door or window, or wear it as a jewelry piece. (Some of these amulets are beautiful artwork). Consecrate it with the following prayer.

Prayer of the Three Nails

The Three Nails and the Cross go before me, Jesus Christ died on it. This cross answers and speaks for me and softens the hearts of those who plot against me. Amen.

Via Crucis: Representation of Stations of the Cross

The via crucis is one of the most popular Good Friday traditions in Mexico. It uses actors to dramatize each of the most important moments of Jesus's life from the way of the cross to the top of Mount Calvary. This staging allows the audience to relive the journey of Jesus to Calvary.

If you do not have a way to participate in one, you can bring to life the spirit of this tradition by watching it on your TV or playing YouTube videos from past year's via crucis.

Good Friday Spell to Recover Something Stolen

There is a myth that the two thieves who ended up on either side of Christ at His crucifixion had a run-in with the Holy Family when Jesus was just an infant, that it was predicted that the thieves would be crucified with Him in Jerusalem, and that Dismas, the penitent thief, would accompany Him to Paradise.

Tradition tells us that Saint Dismas was the good thief who was crucified next to Jesus on Good Friday and is also known as the Good Thief who asked Jesus Christ to remember him in his kingdom. Some Catholics feel that it is not "fair" that Dismas was a criminal who had lived a life of sin and then in his last minutes of life on Earth was saved. They feel that it doesn't seem right that someone could lead their whole life in sin and then be saved at the "last minute," but the Jesus who would save Saint Dismas at the last moment is the one that is believed in and prayed to by brujas de rancho.

There is a very traditional spell that people in the ranchos perform on this day to recover stolen things—even stolen husbands. For this spell, you will need:

> One image of Saint Dismas next to the crucified Christ.
> One piedra imán (lodestone) or magnet
> One pair of cloth gloves, preferably white.
> One white panuelo (handkerchief)

Place your lodestone or magnet on the image of the Good Thief (you can use an image you printed out or a prayer card). Place the image and the lodestone or magnet between both gloves and wrap them with a totally white cloth. Place this inside the drawer of a closet or wardrobe. Do not unwrap the cloth until you recover what was stolen. At the point you place your wrapped bundle in its place, say the following prayer.

The Prayer to the Good Thief

> *Dear Lord, look upon me like you did to the Good Thief. I'm a sinner, already suffering for my faults, but recognizing your divinity. I beg for mercy, strength, and forgiveness. Saint Dismas, I need to be lucky, forgiven, and full of peace as you are. Beside the Beloved One, by ruthless Romans, both of you dead and crucified, I ask you, Good Thief, to bring me back what was stolen, in the name of Jesus Christ. Amen.*

Easter Eve: Holy Saturday

Holy Saturday or Brujas de Rancho's Day? In Mexico, Holy Saturday is an opportunity to cleanse oneself of evil. The Catholic community takes advantage of the day to purify themselves with water and have some fun with it.

One of the most widespread traditions of Holy Week in Mexico is the mythical burning *Quema del Judas*, a life-sized doll representing Judas Iscariot, stuffed with straw and thirty coins. The doll is dressed in clothes donated by people in the rancho. The clothes must have a bad vibe attached to them; either they were worn at funerals or when people had an accident or a breakup. This doll is hung in public and burned in a fervent popular celebration. The public yearly burning is revenge for Judas's betrayal. This tradition varies from place to place, often taking on additional political or spiritual connotation.

This night is when water and fire are blessed in Catholic churches around the world. After this blessing, Easter begins. It is a beautiful night for brujas because it is believed by the faithful that after that day, Jesus Christ showed the world his concrete mission to die and resurrect, the last sacrifice for humanity to free us from sin. It is a magical night where you can feel the energy and the transition. The Saturday of Glory is the day when *brujos y brujas* come out with buckets or pitchers of water to be blessed by the priest.

This night is the best time to get materials to work, such as the paschal candle, Holy Water, salt, and oil. We bless our statues and rosaries and get ready to stay up until very late. The vigil outside the church begins between sunset on Holy Saturday and sunrise on Easter Sunday, when an Easter fire is kindled and the Paschal candle is blessed and then lit. My grandma used to take a basket with a lot of water bottles, three white handkerchiefs, one crucifix, a rosary, three paschal candles, salt, olive oil, dirt, medals, and all the images and statues that she bought during the year. She would place it at the altar, where everyone is doing exactly the same, trying to be discrete. After the vigil, everything that was placed on the altar, such as the entire contents of my grandmother's basket, is considered a sacramental.

To add more power to sympathetic magic, use that blessed paschal candle and Holy Water to baptize your puppets and fetiches.

Personal Judas Spell

On this day, brujas de rancho make their own Judas doll and burn it at 3 PM so they are ready to assist with the paschal vigil during the night. Be aware that this spell is very powerful and dangerous, since at that time not only brujas but also Catholics in general are burning their own Judas all along the Mexican territory. Even though every Judas has a different face, the feelings of hatred are everywhere, and the devils are loose, celebrating for a couple hours that Jesus entered death and stayed dead. The gap is long enough to cause irreparable damages to people who do not protect themselves or are not aware of this kind of practice.

This is not a spell to seek a redress of balance. This is a spiteful vengeance spell, one that will lead your target to hang themselves, physically, spiritually, or financially. The phrase *"[He] went and hanged himself."* (Matt 27:5) can be interpreted literally as an act of suicide. For the tradition, the phrase can be a figurative one: there are a lot of ways we can hang ourselves so be righteous— act and think with a good level of discernment. You will not be working through the Father, you cannot work it with the Son, and no one is able to reach the Holy Spirit on this day. For a couple of hours, evil is all you have.

For this spell, you will need:

A bunch of hate
Your spell scissors
A handmade rag doll
Jute twine string
Thirty coins (the lighter and smaller, the better, and preferably silver color)
A black candle
Matches

You will also need one thing that belongs to your personal Judas Iscariot. You can use hair, nail clippings, or clothes. In case you don't have access to any of their belongings, use a picture of them or introduce a paper with the person's name inside the doll. The goal is to make a sympathetic magic doll; remember that this doll creation is representative of another person, so the more or best personalized items you can use for this, the better it will be. The thread, material, colors, and filling are totally up to you, but I advise to you to dress the doll with material that is similar to what the other person tends to wear, in the same colors or style. Most importantly, it should have something very personal to the other person.

First things first: make your doll. Once you have finished it, you are going to cut open a hole where the anus would be and introduce the thirty coins one by one, saying the name of the person every time you put a coin inside of it. Then you are going to sew it up with the needle and thread. Give the doll a cynical and spiteful kiss, knowing that you are going to burn it. Use the jute twine string to hang it outside in a safe place to burn. Remember that the doll will fall once it is in flames, so for a safer choice, place a pot or flame-resistant container beneath the doll to catch it.

Before you light the doll on fire, repeat the following the prayer:

Lord of lies whose power is absolute tonight. You, who entered
into Judas Iscariot's soul, and infested it with your hatred, with

your envy, with sin and doom. Him, who was one of the twelve dis-
ciples, who was chosen to be among the twelve, one of God's most
trusted companions. But instead, he betrayed with a kiss, and gave
his friend over to torture and certain death in exchange for thirty
pieces of silver.... I beg to you to do the same that you did to Judas
Iscariot to (name of the target). Infest (target's pronouns) with
your most disgusting larvae, so it leads (target's name) to death, I
disown (target's pronouns) three times just like Peter did to Jesus,
his friend. Lead (target's name) to death, this person has already
collected (target's pronouns) thirty pieces of silver, just like the trai-
tor did. I promise not to forget this favor and in return (here make
an offering that is worthy of this favor). Amen.

Domingo de Resurrección: Easter

Easter Sunday is the day that closes the Easter Season, which lasts fifty days
in total, beginning with Easter Sunday and ending on Pentecost Sunday.
This is the Sunday on which Jesus rose from the dead on the third day to
ascend to heaven and be at the right hand of the Father, as the holy scrip-
tures indicate.

Very early in the morning, uncover your holy images that you covered
up on Good Friday. If you dressed your Virgin Mary in black, you must now
put her normal clothes back.

Capirotada

One of the Lenten traditions that we enjoy in Mexico is a dessert called
capirotada. It is a bread pudding made with toasted bolillo, piloncillo, cheese,
cloves, nuts, and raisins. Many of these ingredients are magical ones we
already discussed in Chapter Two: The Bruja's Kitchen.

Several references indicate the existence of capirotada recipes in
the Inquisition archives, linking it to both Mexican Lent traditions and

Passover. However, the exact history is murky. My family is more prone to make it Fridays and Easter Sunday. There are many recipes for this traditional dish, and they tend to vary a lot from family to family. Here is my recipe for capirotada, but you can modify it for your individual tastes and needs. Personally, I like to add banana even though they're not traditional. When I make this at home, I leave out the raisins, an important traditional ingredient, because my son hates them.

Capirotada Recipe

Preparation Time: 30 minutes

Baking Time: 35–45 minutes

Total Time: An hour

Piloncillo Soaking Syrup

8oz. piloncillo

Three cloves

One star anise

4 1/2 cups of water

Three cinnamon sticks

Capirotada

1lb. bolillo

4oz. pecans

2oz. peanuts

2oz. raisins

1oz. grageas (sprinkles)

8oz. cubed queso fresco

To make the soaking syrup, add 4 cups of water, the piloncillo, the cinnamon sticks, cloves, and star anise to a large saucepan. Turn on high, cover, and bring to a boil. Once piloncillo has completely dissolved, turn off and set aside. Remove the cinnamon sticks, cloves, and the star anise from the soaking syrup. You can use a kitchen strainer.

To assemble the capirotada, preheat the oven to 450 degrees. Using a sharp break knife, cut the bolillo in half-inch slices across the center. For an even cut across, put your left hand firmly down on top of the bolillo and with your right hand begin cutting through the middle of the bolillo. Toast the bread in a pan.

In a 9x13 inch baking dish, assemble the layers by first pouring a thin layer of soaking syrup and then proceed with the toasted bread, peanuts, pecans, and cheese. Soak the first layer evenly with the piloncillo syrup. Repeat the layers until all the ingredients have been added. Pour any remaining syrup over the top. Finish by topping with extra peanuts and pecans.

Bake the capirotada at 450 degrees for twenty minutes. Remove the dish from the oven and decorate with raisins and grageas. Let the pudding cool slightly before serving. Capirotada can be served either warm or cold.

MAGICAL CORRESPONDENCE

Brujeria de Rancho is very casual, practical, and easy. Most of the works, spells, and rituals can be practiced at any time, at any place, and using what we have at hand. This type of magic was born from necessity, crises, and lack of resources; it is prepared to be flexible. However, there are certain simple things that will increase and enhance the power of this magic. Just like in many magical traditions, we use what are known as "correspondences" to create magical links. Correspondence tables in Brujeria de Rancho can help you to select colors, days, or hours to use or follow in a ritual or working.

I know you may be wondering, since when did Mexican brujos start working with planetary aspects, moon phases, and correspondences? The answer is that we have for centuries been working our magic this way. This tradition is the result of the mixture of native cultures' beliefs and other contributions that arrived latter.

Take a look at the following lists of magical correspondences and use them when working on spell or ritual constructions of your own.

Velacion/Candle Burning

For those who do not know or have never been able to explain why candles are lit in Mexican Brujeria, the answer is simple: No operation, whether magical or religious, can achieve its mission if the position and the will of the participants is not sealed through a velacion. A velacion is the act of lighting a certain number of candles according to a certain formation, color, shape, and material corresponding to the desired purpose. In the case of Brujeria de Rancho, we limit ourselves to the use of a single candle, sometimes two. Personally, I like to use regular colored spell candles, but if you prefer to use prayer candles or seven day candles in glass (which are safer if you have small kids), you should substitute them. This is totally about availability; use what you have and what you like.

White	Purity, protection, spiritual strength, balance, harmony, communion
Red	Passion, lust, vigor, strength, power, protection, sex, conquering, courage, passionate love
Yellow	Wealth, brightness, wisdom, abundance, blessings, light happiness
Green	Money, possessions, wealth, fortune
Blue	Study, communication, stability, education
Baby Blue	Soothing, cooling, calm
Pink	Friendship, true love, tenderness
Gold	Attraction, magnetic, fortune, alluring, captivating, opulence
Silver	Charity, wealth, spiritual protection, defense
Brown	Court cases, law matters
Orange	Combination of yellow and red, prosperity, good luck
Purple	Psychic ability, Psychic power, spirituality, wisdom, high power, intuition, mysticism
Black	Banishing, harm, destruction of good or bad, death, necromancy

Colors

Work with candles according to the vibratory desire or specific influence symbolized by its color.

Dressing

In Brujeria de Rancho, it is absolutely essential to dress a candle with oil and to impress upon it your desire and intentions. In regard to what oil to use, this is a matter you should decide for yourself. You can use a premade botanica oil, craft your own, or use simple olive oil, which is an all-purpose oil that is very accessible and easy to hide in case you need to disguise your craft. The anointing and the dressing are very simple. We dress the whole candle by anointing it with the oil using your hands from the top to the bottom, or by poking holes in top of candle and dripping oil inside. After you've anointed your candle, sprinkle on the herbs of the working. (Not all candles are meant to be dressed by herbs but all of them should be burned with oil.)

Moon Phases

The notion that shifts in lunar gravitational forces are reflected in agricultural and magical activities has existed for centuries, and it's something to take into consideration to plan our workings. Remember that the dark moon is the roughly three days in which the moon is not visible to us.

Moon Phase	Magic and properties
New moon	New beginnings, fertility, intention setting, renewal
Waxing crescent	Action, things growing, increase
First quarter	Luck spells, road-opener spells
Waxing gibbous	Build, create, gestation, short-term goals
Full moon	Light, abundance, power, love spells
Waning gibbous	Breaking curses, cancel spells
Last quarter	Removals, cleansings, endings
Waning crescent	Rest, limpias, get rid of, let go, dissemination, separation spells
Dark moon	Hexing, banishing, binding hiding, necromancy, divination

Days

Days and hours are important in the practice of Brujeria de Rancho. This correspondence of days and hours to planets is based on the ancient Chaldean astrological system. Each day the week and every hour of the day are ruled by a planet, which gives it a unique energy that will give extra power to your magic. Choosing what day and what hour is best for your planned action is a matter of knowing which planet most favorably corresponds with your intent for that action. For example, if you're doing something secretive, an hour of the Sun is probably the worst hour you could choose. A love spell can make for some interesting hours decisions. If you want to have sex with a person, it could be done in the hour of Venus (for eroticism) on Tuesday (for Mars) because you are focused on the act of sex itself (which is ruled by Mars). This would be a good way to combine the two influences.

Days	Planet	Magic
Sunday	Sun	Everything good under the sun, creativity, enlightenment, success, triumph, honor
Monday	Moon	Home, psychic power, fertility, intuition, emotions, perception, clairvoyance
Tuesday	Mars	Protection, battle, domination, victory, war, courage, action, risk, sex
Wednesday	Mercury	Communication and language, legal, school, commerce, travel (business), career
Thursday	Jupiter	Good fortune, abundance, prosperity, generosity, travel (pleasure), expansion, luck
Friday	Venus	Love, lust, romance, attraction, sensuality, friendship, social relationships, seduction
Saturday	Saturn	Hexing, banishing, authority, binding, defense, necromancy, restriction, death

Hours

Each hour is ruled by a specific planet, and every planet has its own individual characteristics and energy, which clearly show themselves during the associated hour. This method has been used in agriculture, as well as in magic and ritual work, for thousands of years. Along with the lunar calendar, planetary hours are a great way to go even deeper and more specifically into the influence of a day

This method is very specific, and you will need only to follow the next steps to calculate your planetary hours if you intend to calculate them by hand. Today of course you don't *need* to calculate planetary hours by hand, and there are a lot of planetary hour calculators online that will do the math for you.

- *Find out the sunrise and sunset times for your area. (You can use any search engine to get this information.)*

- *Figure out the hour and minute difference between the two times and convert that to minutes.*

- *Convert the sunlight hours into minutes by multiplying the hours by 60 and adding the remaining minutes, then divide by 12. Do the same for night hours, which will be the exact opposite times.*

- *The sunrise time is the start of the first hour.*

- *To find the second hour, and each hour after that, add the planetary hour length to the previous hour time.*

- *Repeat this process until you reach sunset.*

- *Redo this process to find the night hours, consulting the night portion of the chart below, and calculating from sunset of the current day to sunrise of the next day.*

- *This can get a bit confusing because each day is different and there is a lot of math involved. The good news is there is a ton of resources available online or apps you can download that will give you the planetary hours for the current day.*

Use the chart below to find out the planetary rulings for each day. (It is not difficult to find out which planet rules the hour. The first hour of any day is always ruled by the planet which rules that Planetary Day.)

Hours	Sunday	Monday	Tuesday	Wednesday	Thursday	Friday	Saturday
1	Sun	Moon	Mars	Mercury	Jupiter	Venus	Saturn
2	Venus	Saturn	Sun	Moon	Mars	Mercury	Jupiter
3	Mercury	Jupiter	Venus	Saturn	Sun	Moon	Mars
4	Moon	Mars	Mercury	Jupiter	Venus	Saturn	Sun
5	Saturn	Sun	Moon	Mars	Mercury	Jupiter	Venus
6	Jupiter	Venus	Saturn	Sun	Moon	Mars	Mercury
7	Mars	Mercury	Jupiter	Venus	Saturn	Sun	Moon
8	Sun	Moon	Mars	Mercury	Jupiter	Venus	Saturn
9	Venus	Saturn	Sun	Moon	Mars	Mercury	Jupiter
10	Mercury	Jupiter	Venus	Saturn	Sun	Moon	Mars
11	Moon	Mars	Mercury	Jupiter	Venus	Saturn	Sun
12	Saturn	Sun	Moon	Mars	Mercury	Jupiter	Venus
13	Jupiter	Venus	Saturn	Sun	Moon	Mars	Mercury
14	Mars	Mercury	Jupiter	Venus	Saturn	Sun	Moon
15	Sun	Moon	Mars	Mercury	Jupiter	Venus	Saturn
16	Venus	Saturn	Sun	Moon	Mars	Mercury	Jupiter
17	Mercury	Jupiter	Venus	Saturn	Sun	Moon	Mars
18	Moon	Mars	Mercury	Jupiter	Venus	Saturn	Sun
19	Saturn	Sun	Moon	Mars	Mercury	Jupiter	Venus
20	Jupiter	Venus	Saturn	Sun	Moon	Mars	Mercury
21	Mars	Mercury	Jupiter	Venus	Saturn	Sun	Moon
22	Sun	Moon	Mars	Mercury	Jupiter	Venus	Saturn
23	Venus	Saturn	Sun	Moon	Mars	Mercury	Jupiter
24	Mercury	Jupiter	Venus	Saturn	Sun	Moon	Mars

GLOSSARY

Abrecaminos: A plant used for road opening rituals or spells.

Abre caminos: A type of magic whose goal is to open, clear, or create roads, the pathways to a good life full of blessings.

Agua del carmen: A medicinal formula created in 1611 by Discalced Carmelites in order to cure folk illness.

Aguamiel: The sap of the agave plant that is harvested in order to drink fresh or ferment into pulque. Translates to "honey water."

Aguardiente: An alcoholic beverage made from sugar cane. Translates to "fiery water."

Ajo macho: Male garlic.

alum stone: Hard crystalline stone, composed of potassium, aluminum, hydrogen, sulfur, and oxygen. It has antiseptic and spiritual properties.

amarre: A type of working to tie two people together romantically.

amatl: A type of bark paper that was manufactured out of fig trees in Mexico before the conquest. The Spanish word is "amate."

Anima Sola: The spirit of Maria Celestina Abdegano, a soul in pain who is in purgatory. Anima Sola translates to "lonely soul."

Anusim: People who were forced to abandon Judaism against their will after being forcibly converted to Catholicism. The word translates to "coerced."

apostemas: Sores.

bacanora: Traditional drink in the state of Sonora, Mexico, produced from agave Pacifica. Also called Agave Yaquiana.

baños: Spiritual baths or showers.

barro: Mexican clay.

Belzebuth: The prince of demons.

bolillo: Small loaf of plain white bread, crusty on the outside with a soft interior. The French baguette was transformed in Mexico and became the bolillo.

botanica: A Hispanic esoteric shop.

bruja: A Spanish word that translates to witch, it has different meanings and connotations depending on the context and the culture or country where the word is used.

bruja de rancho: A female identified person practicing Brujeria de Rancho. The term is used to refer to individuals who master combinations of brujeria, hechicería, ensalmacion, folk psychology, and necromancy.

brujeria: Formally translates to witchcraft, practice based on pacts with spirits to seek personal gain for ourselves or others.

Brujeria de Rancho: A mixture of Mexican folk practices in rural areas of Mexico.

Brujeria Mexicana: Mexican witchcraft.

brujo: A male identified witch.

cantarito: Handmade pear-shaped jug made from Mexican clay pottery.

capirotada: Mexican bread pudding consumed mostly on Lent.

carniceria: Butcher shop.

catechumen: A Christian convert who has not been baptized.

cedula: A prayer card containing a powerful exorcism.

Cenizo: *Eucophyllum frutescens,* Texas sage, a purple-flowering shrub.

chamuscar: Spanish word meaning "to burn."

chancaca: Rectangular tablet made with honey obtained from sugar cane.

Chantico: Aztec Goddess of the hearth.

Chicomecóatl: Aztec corn goddess.

cibih: Fright in the Zapotec language.

cihuapatli: A name applied to several medicinal plants used to induce contractions during childbirth, or to make a woman experience strong orgasms.

cocolmeca: Used as anti-inflammatory, antiulcer, antioxidant, anticancer, diaphoretic, and for its diuretic properties in northeastern Mexico.

Converso: A Jew who converted to Catholicism in Spain or Portugal.

cordero manso: A meek lamb.

corridos: A music genre with a narrative ballad, usually with accordion, in Mexican rural working-class culture.

Crypto-Judaism: Secret adherence to Judaism while publicly professing to adherence to Christianity. Through generations, this secret can get buried, as many from Crypto-Jewish families have no idea of their heritage.

curandera: A folk healer.

Day of the Dead: A holiday celebrated in Mexico and other Latin American countries to celebrate and honor our deceased people.

dicho: Traditional Mexican saying.s

Ehecatl: Aztec God of Wind.

El Campo Santo: Burial ground.

El Chamuco: El Diablo, the devil.

El Charro Negro: A folk spirit from the Mexican revolution.

empacho: Mexican folk illness, defined as an obstruction of the stomach and/or intestine due a large amount of food or flour, creating a type of very painful indigestion and paralysis of the digestive system.

endulzamiento: Sweetening spell to resolve grievances or arguments between people.

ensalmacion: The act of curing or healing with ensalmos.

ensalmadores: People practicing ensalmacion.

ensalmería: A folk healing practice through words and prayers.

ensalmo: Folk healing prayer or verbal charm.

entierros: Burials.

eschatology: A theology concerned with death, and the final destiny of the soul.

Espiritismo: A doctrine that studies the nature, origin, and destiny of spirits, as well as their cause and effect relationship as a consequence of actions executed in past lives. Spiritism is based on the five books of the Spiritist Codification written by French educator Hypolite Léon Denizard Rivail under the pseudonym Allan Kardec.

Fetiches: Object usually in the form or a shape of a doll that represents a specific person. Used for sympathetic magic.

hamsa: Palm-shaped amulet or talisman popular throughout North Africa and in the Middle East. It is also known as the hand of Fatima and the hand of Miriam.

hechicería: Sorcery.

hechicero: Sorcerer.

hechizos: Spells.

Huapangos: Mexican dance and music genre from the state of Veracruz

huipil: An ancient one-piece garment often decorated with colorful embroidery, it is worn as a blouse or dress by women in Mexico.

Ihiyotl: A Nahuatl word for the animating force that resides within the liver, a luminous gas with odor that only departs from the body in death.

ixtle: a plant fiber used for cordage.

Jabon Zote: Mexican laundry soap.

jícara: A vessel made with the peel of the fruit of the jícara tree.

Justo Juez Negro: The Righteous Black Judge. An invocation of the devil.

jute cord: Low stretch, food-safe, biodegradable twine roping.

Ladino: A dialect of Spanish that developed among Sephardic Jews; the Judeo-Spanish language.

lazo: Rope made of flowers, beads, or other materials, placed around the shoulders of the couple in a Mexican Catholic wedding.

limpias: Spiritual cleansings.

machismo: Aggressive and toxic masculinity.

Macuilxochitl: Aztec God of gambling, dancing, music, sacred ball games, and hemorrhoids.

maleficio: A malediction.

malinalli: Two twisted straws. Also means "to twist."

Mano Ponderosa: The Roman Catholic image of the Powerful Hand.

Mayahuel: Known as "the woman of the 400 breasts," she is the spirit of the maguey plant (*Agave americana*), and also part of a complex of interrelated maternal and fertility goddesses.

mecate: Rope

Mecatlapuhqui: Pre-Hispanic sorceress who healed and did divination through cords.

mestiza/mestizo: A woman or man, respectively, of mixed race.

molcajete: Mexican mortar and pestle made out volcanic rock.

mometzcopinqui: A term for women born on the date of Ce-Ehecatl (meaning "One-wind" or "One-rain"), a pre-Hispanic witch.

momochtli: Pre-Hispanic popcorn.

morralitos: A cotton or rayon fabric bag used to contain Mexican spiritual amulets.

muñecos: Dolls.

Nahuatl: An Aztecan language family.

nazar: A powerful amulet used for protection against the Evil Eye; also known as the *ojo turco* in Spanish.

novena: Special prayers that last nine days.

ocote: *Pinus montezumae,* a conifer in the family *Pinaceae.* It has cleansing and protective powers in Mexican Folklore.

ofrendas: Offerings.

ombliguera: An obsidian navel stone.

piedra imán: Lodestone.

piloncillo: Raw form of pure cane sugar that is commonly used in Mexican cooking, sometimes referred to as Mexican brown sugar. It is called panela in other Latin American countries.

rancheras: A genre of traditional music in Mexico.

ranchitos: A group of ranches, the plural of ranch.

rancho: Ranch.

resguardos: A type of protections put in place to protect a person or a family household.

sacrament: Catholic rite.

sacramentals: Object or action blessed by a Catholic priest.

Sahumar: To clean through smoke, to flood a place or space with smoke. This practice consists of burning herbs, resins, woods, powders, or flowers on lit charcoal or a bundle in a bowl suitable for high temperatures.

Sahumerio: Aromatic smoke that can be made from herbs, resins, wood, flowers, and other materials.

salación: A type of working to make a person, business, or household become financially bankrupt and unemployable, so that they cannot prosper in any aspect related to money. Salacións can also be used to make someone romantically unlovable, sick, or all of the above.

salaciónes: Different kinds or varieties of salación workings, the plural of salación.

salado/salada: An extremely negative and unpleasant mental, financial, physical, moral, and spiritual state.

susto: A fright or scare; a spiritual illness that results from a sudden fright.

tilma: An ancient one-piece garment often decorated with colorful embroidery worn by men in Mexico.

Tlaloc: Aztec God of rain, water, lightning, and agriculture.

Tlaloques: Tlaloc's (the Aztec God of Rain) little helpers.

Tlatlauhqui-cihuatl-ichilzintli: Respectable lady of the red chile.

Tlazolteotl: Goddess of Cotton, Goddess of Filth, Goddess of Birth.

Tlazolteotl-Ixcuina: Goddess of Cotton.

tonalli: Part of the soul, located in the crown of the head, that regulated body temperature and played a major role in determining a person's destiny.

trabajo: Spiritual spell intended to harm, dominate, or control someone.

Tzitzimimeh: Lesser deities associated with the stars, depicted as skeletal female figures.

velacion: The act of lighting candles according to certain formations and times, which correspond to a desired purpose.

Via crucis: The Stations of the Cross, commemorating Jesus's passion and death on the cross.

Vueltas: Circular laps.

zoapatle: *Montanoa tomentosa,* a species of flowering plant.

BIBLIOGRAPHY

Argüelles, Gabriel Ignacio Verduzco. *The Oral Tradition on Witchcraft in the Southeast of the State of Coahuila: Language, Contexts and Symbolic Production.* Dissertation. *www.academia.edu.*

Báez-Jorge, F. *Los Oficios de las Diosas Xalapa.* Universidad Veracruzana. 1988.

Campos Moreno, Araceli. *Oraciones, Ensalmos y Conjuros Mágicos del Archivo Inquisitorial de la Nueva España.* Campos (El Colegio de México) 2001.

Carranza Vera, Claudia. *La Ascensión y la Caída Diablos: Brujas y Posesas en México y Europa.* (El Colegio de San Luis, México) 2013.

Castaneda, Laura. "La Petaca Witches." *Los Angeles Times,* 1991. *www.latimes.com.*

Chava Halevy, Schulamith. *Descendants of the Anusim in Contemporary Mexico.* (Hebrew University) 2009.

Coltman, Jeremy D. and John M.D Pohl. *Sorcery in Mesoamerica.* (University Press Colorado) 2021.

De la Serna, Jacinto. Manual de Ministros de Indios para el Conocimiento de Sus Idolatrias y Extirpacion de Ellas. (Imprenta de la Museo Nacional) 1656.

El Ritmo de las Oraciones, Ensalmos y Conjuros Mágicos Novohispanos 1600-1630 Edición Anotada y Estudio Preliminar. (Facultad de Filosofía y Letras UNAM) 1994.

Eugenia Flores, María and Gabriel Ignacio Verduzco. *La Producción Ficcional de los Hablantes del Noreste de México: La Simbólica de las Doce Verdades del Mundo.* (Universidad Autónoma de Nuevo León UANL) 2013.

Encausse, Dr. G. *El Embrujamiento.* Papús (Ediciones del más allá) 1932.

García Ávila, Celene, *Amuletos, Conjuros y Pócimas de Amor: Un caso de Hechicería Juzgado por el Santo Oficio* (Puebla de los Ángeles 1652) (Contribuciones desde Coatepec UNAM) 2009.

Gil Olmos, José. *Santos Populares: La fe en Tiempos de Crisis.* (Penguin Random House Grupo Editorial) 2016.

Hacks, Dr. Hector. *Libro Negro:Tratado de Ciencias Ocultas.* (Edicomunicacion S.A.) 1992.

Illes, Judika. *Encyclopedia of Mystics, Saints, and Sages.* (HarperOne) 2011.

Isasi-Diaz, Ada Maria and Fernando F. Segovia, Eds. *Hispanic/Latino Theology: Challenge and Promise.* 1996.

La Brujeria en el México Antiguo: Comentario Crítico en Dimensión Antropológica, vol. 4, mayo-agosto 1995, pp.7-36.

Lévy, Issac Jack and Rosemary Lévy Zumwalt. *Ritual Medical Lore of Sephardic Woman: Sweetening the Spirits, Healing the Sick.* Board of Trustees of the University of Illinois, 2002.

Ligia, Rivera Domínguez. *La bruja Mometzcopinqui, Reina de la Noche.* (Escritos, Revista del Centro de Ciencias del Lenguaje, Numero 22, Julio-diciembre de 2000, pp. 53-94)

López, Austin Alfredo. *Tres Recetas Para un Aprendiz de Mago.* (Ojarasca) 1993.

Madsen, William and Claudia. *A Guide to Mexican Witchcraft.* (Minutiae Mexicana, S.A. de C.V.) 1999.

Masera, Mariana, and Araceli Campos Moreno. *Ensalmos Novohispanos, Palabras Mágicas para Curar, La Otra Nueva España la Palabra Marginada en la Colonia.* (Azul Editorial, UNAM) 2002.

Olmos, Jose Gil. *Los Bruos del Poder: El Occultismo en la Política Mexicana.* Mondadori, Random House, 2007.

Pactum, la Obra Magistral de la Hechicería Antigua. Colección Ciencias Ocultas (Editorial Caymi publicidad ateneo) 1957.

Pocurull, Joaquin. *Extractos de la Leyenda de Colorados de Abajo.* 2020.

Randolph, L. F. "New Evidence on the Origin of Maize." The American Naturalist, vol. 86, no. 829, 1952

Reyes Nolasco, José. Cuextécatl Volvió a la Vida"(Historia, leyendas y costumbres huastecas - 2000)

Rossell, Cecilia and Maria de los Angeles Ojeda Diaz. *Women and Their Goddesses in the Pre-Hispanic Codices of Oaxaca.* CIESAS, 2003.

Santos, Richard G. *Silent Heritage: The Sephardim and the Colonization of the Spanish North American Frontier 1492-1600.* New Sepharad Press, 2000.

Scheffler, Lilian. *Magia y Brujeria en México.* (Panorama Editorial S.A. de C.V.) 1999.

Semboloni, Lara. *Cacería de Brujas en Coahuila 1748-1751 De Villa en Villa sin Dios ni Santa María.* (El Colegio de México) 2003.

Solange, Alberro. *Inquisición y Sociedad en México 1571-1700.* (Fondo de Cultura económica) 1988.

Sufurino, Jonas *El libro de San Cipriano: Libro Completo de Verdadera Magia, o Sea, Tesoro del Hechicero.* (Editorial Maxtor) 2014.

Sullivan, T. *Tlazolteotl-Ixcuina: The Great Spinner and Weaver. The Art and Iconography of Late Post-Classic Mexico.* Elizabeth Hill Boone, Ed. Dumbarton Oaks, Washington DC, 1977.

Vicente, Castro (A.C. Arquivo) *El libro de San Cipriano y Santa Justina: Y Oraciones de la S.S. Cruz de Caravaca.* Tratado Completo para Ejercitar el Poder Oculto. (Edición blanco y . . . de los Libros Maravillosos) 2020.

ABOUT THE AUTHOR

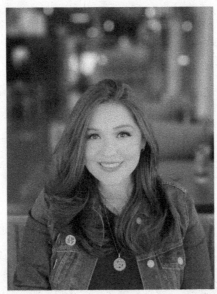

Photo by Scott Ihrig

Laura Davila, a.k.a. Daphne la Hechicera, is a fifth-generation Mexican witch, a long-time practitioner of Mexican ensalmeria, hechicería, brujeria and folk Catholicism. She learned her practice at her grandmothers' knees. Born and raised in Mexico, Laura has lived in the United States since about 2010. Laura identifies as a "bruja de rancho"—a "ranch witch"—a term with great resonance in Mexico indicating knowledge of botanicals and the natural world. Laura is also a Tarot card reader and a flower essence practitioner. Follow her on Instagram @daphne_la_hechicera.

ABOUT THE AUTHOR

TO OUR READERS